HYPNOTIC METHODS IN NONHYPNOTIC THERAPIES

HYPNOTIC METHODS IN NONHYPNOTIC THERAPIES

AARON NOAH HOORWITZ, Ph.D.

IRVINGTON PUBLISHERS, INC.
740 Broadway
New York, New York 10003

Library of Congress Cataloging-in-Publication Data

Hoorwitz, Aaron Noah.
　　Hypnotic methods in nonhypnotic therapies.

　　Bibliography: p.
　　Includes index.
　　1. Hypnotism—Therapeutic use. 2. Hypnotism—
Therapeutic use—Case studies. I. Title. [DNLM:
1. Hypnosis—methods. WM 415 H789h]
RC497.H66 1989　　　616.89'14　　　　　　87-31046
ISBN 0-8290-1802-6

10 9 8 7 6 5 4 3 2 1

Printed in the United States of America

The paper used in this publication meets the minimum requirements of American National Standard for Information Sciences—Permanence of Paper for Printed Library Materials, ANSI Z39.48-1984.

CONTENTS

ACKNOWLEDGMENTS

I am grateful to a number of individuals for their helpful comments, criticisms, and suggestions on earlier drafts of this manuscript, especially John J. O'Connor, Lisa L. Adams, and Anthony Gaito.

Special thanks are due to John O'Connor for providing the FORE-WORD to this manuscript, for thought-provoking discussions which helped in the writing of it, and for his encouragement and support. I am particularly indebted to Lisa Adams, a master of the double bind, for helping me to better learn to think on my feet while navigating my way through the subtle web of paradoxical communications. I also thank my mother, Marion Hoorwitz, for providing me, in my earliest years, with a great deal of first hand experience in the artful use of hypnotic ritual; this experience has helped me to better understand, apply, and explain uses of ritual.

It is also important to me to respectfully acknowledge the wisdom of many sources whose ideas appear in this work and who have influenced my understanding of therapy. There are too many to fully enumerate here. They include those whose ideas are well known in the field of psychotherapy, such as Jay Haley, Gregory Bateson, Milton Erickson, and Cloe Madanes, as well as those outside of the field, such as Jose Ortega y Gasset, William Shakespeare, and Lau Tsu.

Finally, I am grateful for the questions asked by students and by therapists who have struggled to understand and to integrate hypnotic methods in their approaches to therapy. It was these questions which led me to believe that there was a need for a book of this kind. This book is a response to those questions.

FOREWORD

When I first met Aaron Hoorwitz 14 years ago in graduate school, he was a young man who approached me one day to discuss and share his excitement in some research he was doing. Unlike anyone else in the department, he was investigating cognitive-developmental stages of humor appreciation. As I think about that time and about his zest, I realize he has always been interested in the unexpected: in incongruities, uses of humor, play, storytelling, metaphor, paradox, and multiple levels of communication. Over the years, he has become one of the best clinician-teachers I know. In his research and teaching, he has struggled to make clear the intricacies and ''logic'' of analogic thought. His left side always understands what the right side is doing. This makes for a thoughtful and balanced therapist and teacher, who has written a thoughtful and lively book.

Aaron's interest in and acceptance of what appears on the surface to be logical contradiction or paradox reminds me of the universal motif in myth and legend regarding the ''coincidence of opposites,'' described by Joseph Campbell in *The Hero with a Thousand Faces*. Opposites or polarities, such as being and not being, life and death, change and stability, are described as the ''clashing of rocks that crush the travelor,'' but between which the heroes must pass. The twin heroes of a Navaho legend were warned of the same obstacle by a figure called the Spider Woman, but were protected by an eagle feather plucked from a living sunbird. I think that therapists are the sons and daughters of Spider Woman and that this book is an eagle feather.

This book is about the use of paradox and polarities. Beginning therapists soon discover that clients usually convey opposite or paradoxical messages, such as ''I want to change, but I can't change'', or ''Please try to change me, but I don't think you can.'' Despite the therapist's best efforts, eloquence, and compassion, change is often difficult to effect. Resolution of this dilemma forms the focal point of many psychotherapies of change, ranging from psychoanalysis to family therapy.

In the Bateson Project, which produced the theory of the double bind, we at last had a beginning understanding, in communication theory, of

vii

the ways in which people qualify and disqualify their messages to others. It gave us more formal ways to describe the paradoxical stance of a client or family who requests change but seems on the surface to resist it. This work resulted in the development of therapeutic paradox to address the problems of clients who are ambivalent about change. Paradoxical approaches can be seen in the works of the Mental Research Institute, Mara Selvini Palazzoli and her associates in Milan, Haley, Madanes, as well as various representatives of the Ackerman Institute.

The approaches described above were also influenced by the hypnotic and "strategic" work of Milton Erickson, which was described over twenty years ago in various publications by Jay Haley. Explicating Erickson's work and using Bateson's communicational terminology, Haley described trance in interactional terms and proposed an equivalence between trance (e.g., "my arm lifts, but not on purpose"), symptomatic complaints (e.g., "I want to change, but I can't"), and therapeutic change (e.g., "I did it, but I'm not sure how"). These equivalences have been difficult to understand in practical contexts but have stimulated exciting strategic and paradoxical approaches to therapy and have encouraged therapists to master hypnotic skills.

However, Haley's work has resulted mainly in making a theoretical point rather than demonstrating how hypnotic and paradoxical methods are inherent in almost every therapy session. Also, the teachings of Erickson and his disciples have tended to be analogical, which makes it somewhat difficult for nonhypnotic therapists to apply hypnotic methods, or to see their relevance, in the everyday practice of therapy. The outcome is that family therapists, as well as other types of therapists, have had some difficulty in integrating hypnotic methods in a general therapeutic practice. Study of Erickson's approach have left many therapists more confused than they were before, more idealizing of Erickson's magic than capable of using it, and more likely to separate hypnotic therapy from brief family or strategic therapy.

Even strategic therapists, whose methods derive in part from a hypnotic approach, often describe cases where they began with or discarded the use of hypnosis and then utilized a "strategic" therapy, as if they were separate types of skills. After reading this book, it is difficult to view hypnotic methods as distinct from the general conduct of therapy. Like Haley, Aaron believes that most therapy is paradoxical and that the hypnotic relationship is essential to any viable therapeutic relationship.

Brief and strategic therapists may recognize hypnotic principles in formulating interventions, but they may be unaware of the hypnotic relationship that is developing between therapist and client or how to maintain consciously a more powerful position of defining the type of therapeutic relationship moment by moment. Aaron's book expands on Haley's theoretical propositions and describes the peculiar form of this interaction in a clear and understandable way so that it can be observed in family therapy or other types of therapy which are not usually considered to be hypnotic, as well as in therapeutic interactions that are more recognizable as hypnotic. His work provides a coherent theoretical and pragmatic link between hypnotic interactions, trance phenomena, and change in any type of therapy.

He repeatedly demonstrates, with specific examples, the equivalence between induction of hypnotic responses and the operations that therapists employ in various nonhypnotic contexts. In doing so, he provides the reader with more consistent ways of conducting therapy so that the reader can see how it is possible to maintain the paradoxical position characteristic of the hypnotic relationship. The therapist's paradoxical position in relation to the client or family's paradoxical challenge is necessarily a fluid one, requiring shifts in how and in what ways the therapeutic relationship is defined. Aaron provides for the reader an intimate understanding of these shifts.

He also clearly describes how the establishment of this kind of therapeutic relationship results in a changing relationship between client and problem or between client and aspects of self or change in the client's view of reality. That is to say, he describes how change is dependent on the kind of therapeutic relationship that is established. This is in the best tradition of Gregory Bateson, who viewed systems or relationship patterns as existing within as well as between people.

The second half of this book is simply delightful to read. By means of 16 brief and extensive case illustrations, Aaron provides wide and creative applications of the theoretical principles outlined in Part I. The cases involve a unique and provocative intervention for smoking, use of ritual to eliminate headache pain in the case of a friend requesting immediate relief, a fascinating and creative treatment in a family therapy session of a child with auditory hallucinations and suicidal ideation, treatment of a woman obsessed with an ex-lover, and interventions for eating disorders, temper tantrums, and a problem of impotence in a couple. There is also a charming and instructive example of a minor therapy "failure". The reader will enjoy the remaining cases as well.

The range of problems treated here reflect the diversity which a therapist in general practice can expect. Yet, each intervention, whether it has the appearance of a strategic intervention, a behavioral method, or any other therapy form, operationalizes the same hypnotic principles. The diversity of the cases permits us to observe these same principles in various contexts, some in which we could easily see the relevance of hypnosis but also some in which we might not imagine hypnotic methods to be relevant to effective therapy.

For example, in one case example, Aaron illustrates the application of hypnotic methods in a nonverbal intervention with a severely retarded adolescent and is able to articulate the equivalence of the interaction to that which occurs in other case illustrations, even in a hypnotic arm levitation. He is able to articulate the equivalence between these forms of interaction and that used in child custody mediation where one might never expect hypnotic principles to have relevance. Case illustrations like these can suggest to hypnotherapists the vast range of applications available for their methods and can suggest to nonhypnotic therapists how an understanding of the hypnotic and paradoxical relationship inherent in most therapy can enhance their usual practices.

By virtue of the diversity of cases illustrated, what stands out is the exact nature of the hypnotic relationship, which is operationalized in every case to provide an invariant sequence of interactions which constitute a vibrant therapeutic relationship. One can observe the way in which various forms of therapy, strategic, behavioral, hypnotic, or otherwise, can fulfill the same identifiable functions in establishing this peculiar form of interaction between therapist and clients and one can see clearly how this form of interaction effects change. One ceases to think of hypnotic methods or the hypnotic relationship as an exotic or specialized approach but rather as a way of thinking about how to conduct good therapy in general.

Aaron's scholarship is evident not just in his familiarity with various forms of therapy, but also in his ready allusions to various analogic traditions. That is, not only does he quote Haley, Erickson, Bateson, and other luminaries in the fields of family, strategic, and hypnotic therapies, but also frequently alludes to Shakespeare, Sun Tzu, Lau Tsu, the Bible, Buddha, shamans, rabbis, and other descendants of the Spider Woman. In doing so, he suggests ways in which various psychological, philosophical, mystical, and cultural traditions are compatible with one another. These allusions hint at a broader understanding about living in harmony with oneself and other things, as well as a way of understanding therapeutic change.

Aaron's writing style may appear to be deceptively simple because he describes extremely complex issues in a way that is clear and straightforward enough to provide guidance to therapists unfamiliar with hypnotic or paradoxical issues. While his view can be regarded as essentially "strategic", since the several strategic approaches are extensions of the model he articulates, he strives to make clear that most other forms of therapy can be used effectively within this model. In no way does he take a chauvinistic position which would attempt to derogate the value of alternate methods of therapy.

Aaron has written a book that will be useful to hypnotherapists who wish to extend their skills to other types of therapy work, but especially to nonhypnotic therapists who wish to utilize hypnotic methods in a manner that is consistent within their own approaches. I look forward to other eagle feathers from this talented man.

John J. O'Connor, Ph.D.

PART 1

THEORETICAL
RATIONALE

1

OVERVIEW

Observers are often impressed by hypnotists who induce trances by uttering what appears to be a casual remark, or by gazing at the subject in a special way, or by telling a story, or even by shaking the subject's hand in such a way that the hand remains extended in the air. Inductions of this kind challenge the popular view of hypnosis as a special state of consciousness which can only be induced by standard and special procedures. Most noticeably, these trance inductions lack direct suggestions for the subject to experience trance. They illustrate an indirect approach to hypnosis which has evolved over the past few decades due in large measure to the influence of Milton Erickson.

In the past several years, an abundant literature has bourgeoned to describe and explain the practice of this indirect hypnotic approach (e.g., Bandler & Grinder, 1975; Erickson, 1983, 1980; Erickson, Rossi & Rossi, 1976; Lankton & Lankton, 1982; Zeig, 1982, 1980). However, use of hypnotic methods in therapeutic situations in which subjects do not expect to experience trance have received only scant treatment in the literature despite the fact that Erickson used hypnotic methods in this way with increasing frequency in the latter stages of his career. The description and explanation of this kind of application of hypnotic methods have usually been insufficient to guide practitioners in successful replications and adaptations to different contexts.

As a consequence, there is still an aura of mystery attached to indirect applications of hypnotic methods. This quality of mystery and the absence of explication, even in literature intended to provide explication and to strip hypnosis of its mystery, serves to unnecessarily befuddle therapists who are struggling to understand and master an indirect hypnotic approach.

Purposes

One of the several purposes of this book is to reduce the mystery attached to indirect uses of hypnotic methods. This purpose will be accomplished by providing an explication of these methods in language which is specific and with examples which are concrete and complete enough to illustrate exactly how these methods are applied in various therapeutic contexts. The focus is not so much on the topic of indirect hypnosis, which has been adequately treated in many other publications, conferences and workshops, as it is on the skills and operations available to the therapist. The aim is to clearly articulate the nature of these skills and some of the specific ways they can be applied in practice so that they are available for adaptation to the reader's own circumstances.

The primary subject of the book does not concern indirect inductions in which the subject expects trance to occur. As was just noted, an abundant literature already exists on this topic. The topic which receives primary attention here concerns situations in which subjects do not necessarily expect to experience trance. In most of these situations, subjects usually remain unaware that trances have occured because the trances are mild ones. From an observer's standpoint, it is not even relevant in some of these instances to determine whether or not a trance can be said to have occured. What is relevant is the way in which hypnotic methods are employed to effect some therapeutic change. Since these methods can be employed in either a hypnotherapeutic context or in a therapeutic context which is not ordinarily associated with hypnosis, a major purpose of the book is to show how hypnotic methods can be effectively used in almost any therapeutic situation.

One way of showing this is by examples which illustrate the application of methods and principles commonly associated with hypnosis in types of therapy which are not normally considered hypnotic therapies. This is the usual form of explication in the literature; it consists of the borrowing of hypnotic methods by nonhypnotic therapies for some circumscribed clinical purpose. Another way of showing how hypnotic methods can be applied in most therapy is from a somewhat opposite point of view, the view that all therapy is essentially hypnotic therapy. A clear recognition of this view can help to guide a therapist's behavior in ways which maximize the impact of therapy regardless of the specific type of therapy, be it behavioral, psychodynamic, strategic, gestalt, or anything else. Both points of view are taken here because each provides a separate perspective of the same therapeutic phenomena; together they facilitate a resonant understanding of these phenomena.

A major stumbling block in the articulation of indirect hypnotic methods in the literature is that the hypnotic methods chosen for examination are usually those which in hypnotherapy are used in the service of convincing subjects that they have been in trances. These methods are usually defined and described in such a way that they seem to belong to the class of exotic and special methods commonly identified with hypnosis. The applications of these methods are usually for circumscribed purposes and also appear exotic, retaining the aura of "hypnosis" as it is commonly understood. Therefore, from this point of view, it is impossible to perceive with clarity the equivalence between an arm levitation with the subject's eyes closed and a family therapy session in which nothing appears to be happening which is usually associated with hypnosis.

This equivalence is easy to see when one realizes that it is not always necessary to convince clients or observers that trance has occured in order to effectively apply hypnotic methods. Many of the facets of a multifaceted hypnotic method are devoted to convincing someone of the existence of a trance and are simply not necessary when there is no need or intent to induce a convincing trance. When the essence of that method is then used in a therapy session, it may go unrecognized as a hypnotic method and simply be considered "good therapy." This is not to say that it is never important to convince clients that they are in a trance. It is often important for various therapeutic purposes; and when it is important, the therapist can avail him or herself of any of the direct or indirect hypnotic techniques that have evolved over the centuries. Yet, for the majority of therapists in the majority of their cases, it is not necessary to convince either the client or observers that the client is in a trance in order to apply hypnotic methods to effect positive change.

Since the view taken here is that almost all therapy is essentially hypnotic, it will be important to show how various therapeutic methods from diverse forms of therapy serve certain hypnotic functions. These functions comprise a conceptual skeletal structure which can guide the use of a variety of therapeutic methods which have evolved throughout history, some of which are associated with the tradition of hypnosis and some of which are not. When this structure of hypnotic functions is made evident, the equivalence between a family therapy session and a behavioral treatment and a hypnotic arm levitation also becomes evident. From this point of view, most moments of almost any therapy session, regardless of the type of therapy, are occasions in which hypnotic methods are being applied more or less successfully.

The focus, then, is on the application of hypnotic methods in the context of a general therapeutic practice in which behavioral, psycho-dynamic, strategic, or any other methods might be employed and in which clients do not necessarily expect to be put into a trance. The book is intended for a readership of general practitioners who wish to sensibly integrate hypnotic methods into their repertoire of existing therapeutic skills. It is not intended to teach the student of hypnosis to induce the impressive trances noted at the beginning of the chapter, for example, inducing a trance by shaking someone's hand in a special way, or by a piercing gaze, or by telling a story. These are the experiences which either client or therapist is convinced are trance experiences and about which a great deal has already been said by many others. Yet, since these applications are merely extensions of the applications which are the main topic of this book, some explanation and description of these forms of induction is inescapable even if only by implication and by illustration of various hypnotic methods.

This differentiation between the general use of hypnotic methods and the use of hypnotic methods to produce a convincing trance is a somewhat arbitrary one, intended only to delimit the primary topic of the book and not at all intended to derogate the use of methods intended to convince someone that trance has occured. In fact, it is hoped that this book will be useful to any type of therapist who employs hypnotic methods, whether it be a traditional hypnotherapist, an Ericksonian hypnotherapist, or a therapist unfamiliar with methods of trance induction and who does not yet know that he or she has probably already been using hypnotic methods.

Organization of the Book

In order to acquaint the general practitioner with those concepts commonly associated with hypnosis, the following chapter is devoted to a brief description of the history of hypnosis, the characteristics which are considered to be its distinguishing features, and a sampling of theories which have been formulated to account for it. The last part of the chapter articulates my own understanding of hypnosis so that the reader can readily differentiate between mine and other theoretical positions.

Chapter Three identifies the general methods and principles commonly associated with hypnosis which are used to induce trance and illustrates by specific examples some ways in which these can be used in nonhypnotic therapies. The intent of these illustrations is to show exactly how hypnotic methods can be employed to induce unexpected trances of which the client remains unaware. As noted above, it is not necessary for either therapist or client to be convinced that trance has occured, but the illustrations are framed with the intent to produce trance so that the extension from commonly known hypnotic methods will be clear and evident; they do not reflect actual intents to "trick" anyone into an undesired trance.

In Chapters Four and Five, a viewpoint is taken which contrasts with but supplements the viewpoint taken in Chapter Three. This is the view which regards most therapy as hypnotic in nature and which relegates specific hypnotic techniques and methods to the same status as specific methods from any form of therapy. These chapters are crucial to an understanding of the others because they provide a unified framework in which one can sensibly use a hypnotic approach in any therapy, or, alternatively, find ways to fine-tune any form of therapy by recognizing and maximizing the ways in which it serves hypnotic functions. The essential hypnotic functions are derived from an understanding of the peculiarities of the hypnotic relationship, which is described in detail in these two chapters. The peculiar form of this relationship constitutes a model for an effective therapeutic relationship in any type of therapy. These chapters show how the establishment of such a relationship creates an optimal interpersonal context for facilitating therapeutic change.

PART 2 of the book consists of case illustrations of hypnotic methods employed in various contexts which are not usually associated with hypnosis. Yet, the degree of association with hypnosis varies from case to case. Most of the cases are elaborated in detail to provide a microscopic focus on both the hypnotic methods being employed and on the methods not usually associated with hypnosis in order to permit the reader to clearly perceive the ways in which methods are integrated with one another. However, the last chapter in this section takes a more distant focus in order to briefly describe numerous case illustrations. The·various case illustrations throughout the chapters sometimes emphasize the ways in which standard hypnotic methods are applied for the purposes of producing certain hypnotic effects, and sometimes emphasize the ways in which all therapy fulfills hypnotic functions. The latter viewpoint, expressed in Chapter Four, is deliberately and exhaustively operationalized in a casette recording for the problem of smoking, a transcript of which appears in the first chapter of PART 2.

The therapist was myself in almost all case illustrations. I will interchangeably refer to myself in the first person, or as the author, or as the therapist, depending on which designation seems most appropriate at each point and depending on which best helps to differentiate between myself and other persons involved in various illustrations. The pronouns "he" and "she" will both be used together to refer to human beings, but when it is cumbersome to use them together, either pronoun by itself may sometimes be used strictly for the sake of stylistic convenience.

As noted earlier, the following chapter is intended primarily for therapists who are unfamiliar with hypnosis. If the reader already possesses familiarity with the history of hypnosis, its characteristics, and theories which attempt to account for it, then I suggest that the reader skip to the last section of the chapter entitled A WORKING DEFINITION OF HYPNOSIS. This section will acquaint the reader with the particular view of hypnosis reflected throughout the book.

2

BACKGROUND AND THEORY

This chapter describes the theoretical and historical context in which the topics of this book are embedded. To provide the widest of perspectives, the chapter begins with a brief discussion of the history of hypnosis. This is followed by characteristics frequently associated with hypnosis, theories formulated to account for it, and the author's theoretical understanding of hypnosis.

History

Hypnotic-like methods have been used throughout history in almost all cultures for both religious and healing purposes (Kroger, 1977). For example, trance inducing techniques appear to have been used by old testament prophets, by Jesus and his disciples, by practitioners of the Jewish mystical tradition of Cabala, by Mohamed, and by Sufi healers (Bowers & Glasner, 1958; Glasner, 1955; Hallaji, 1962). Tribal medicine men, shamans, Egyptian soothsayers, Taoist priests, Persian magi, Indian yogis, religious leaders, and faith healers of various kinds have all recognized the occurence of trance and have employed a variety of trance inducing procedures.

It has only been in the past two hundred years that the concept of "hypnosis" has been used in Western culture to describe trance experiences. Made famous in Europe by Mesmer, trance was first referred to as artificial somnambulism, animal magnetism, and mesmerism; shortly afterward, it was given the name of "hypnotism" by Braid (1843), a Scottish physician, and has been known by this name ever since.

Although the occurence of trance has been recognized, and even deliberately facilitated, for thousands of years, "hypnosis" is a term of relatively recent coinage and refers more to a historical phenomenon than to the experience of trance itself. It refers to the specific methods which evolved to induce it, the therapeutic lore surrounding it, and the cultural myths which have emerged since the time of Mesmer and which do not necessarily serve to define and explain trance phenomena occuring outside this tradition.

For more detailed discussions of early developments in hypnosis and for reviews of the work of the early pioneers in the field, such as Mesmer, Braid, Charcot, Bernheim, and others, the interested reader can consult numerous other sources (e.g., Ellenberger, 1970; Thornton, 1976; Tinterow, 1970). The practice and study of hypnosis in the last hundred and fifty years can be characterized, perhaps in oversimplified terms, as falling into three main approaches: an authoritative and ritualistic approach, an empirical approach, and the Ericksonian approach of indirect suggestion.

The authoritative approach. Formal rituals and authoritative suggestion marked the use of hypnosis from the middle of the 19th century to the middle of the present century. Since hypnosis was viewed for a time as a form of sleep, the practice of this approach frequently included direct suggestions for the subject to go into a deep sleep and hypnosis soon came to be defined by the techniques used to produce it.

This traditional approach has left a stereotyped image of hypnosis in the lay as well as professional mind, which still lingers today. The stereotype is due partly to the frequent use by hypnotists of standard and ritualistic induction procedures which directly request that the subject "sleep" or "relax." It is also due to the fact that a small proportion of individuals are able to achieve a deep somnambulistic trance with apparent ease. These individuals possess a number of common characteristics (Gibson & Corcoran, 1975; Hilgard, 1965, 1970; Lang & Lazowik, 1962), including the possession of an unusually vivid imagination, and can easily experience the more dramatic hypnotic phenomena, such as amnesia and hallucination. Since hypnotists have tended to use these individuals whenever possible for demonstration purposes, the hypnotic capacities and unique experiences of this special population of individuals have fostered a view of hypnotic trance which has been misapplied as a standard for the general population.

The empirical approach. An empirical approach was taken in the study of hypnosis as early as the 1880's by Bernheim and Liebault (Tinterow,

1970). However, it was not until the 1950's that major research efforts were undertaken, sustained by ample federal funding of several research centers in the United States. As a result, diverse aspects of hypnosis have been subjected to experimental scrutiny and a large body of informative research findings has emerged. However, another consequence of the empirical approach was the emergence of the construct of hypnotizability.

In order to study hypnotic phenomena in measurable forms, this approach required standardization of tests of hypnotic susceptibility and of induction procedures. Standardization requires that individuals conform, or be responsive, to a standard set of stimuli, despite the fact that some individuals might be more responsive to nonstandard stimuli. As a consequence, the empirical approach fostered a widely held view that individuals can be characterized by variable degrees of hypnotizability (e.g., Weitzenhoffer & Hilgard, 1959). According to this view, a certain proportion of the population cannot be hypnotized, another proportion can be hypnotized to mild levels of depth, and other proportions can be hypnotized to increasingly greater levels of depth.

The indirect approach. At about the same time that this flurry of research was occuring, Milton Erickson was actively engaged in the practice of hypnosis and in the reformulation of traditional ideas concerning hypnotic methods. He gradually developed an approach that has revolutionized the practice of hypnosis. In Erickson's approach, there is less reliance on standardized techniques and more emphasis placed on an innovative utilization of the subject's unique experiences and responses. Trance is sometimes produced in a very slow and gradual fashion, with a keen sensitivity to, and utilization of, the subject's most subtle responses. This sensitivity to the subject's responses results in a synchrony between hypnotist and subject which is a distinguishing feature of the approach. There is also recognition of the mutuality of influence between hypnotist and subject, with the subject influencing the hypnotist's responses as well as the reverse. The mutuality and synchrony which is established reflect an emphasis on the importance of the hypnotic relationship. Authoritative commands and pressure on the subject to experience trance, while effective in some cases, are usually considered to be unnecessary. For this reason, and because hypnotic methods are often applied indirectly and flexibly, the approach is frequently referred to as indirect hypnosis.

An important implication of the approach is that many people can be hypnotized who show a low degree of hypnotic susceptibility as measured by standardized tests. Tests and standardized induction procedures are not tailored to the unique capacities of individuals, but the indirect approach emphasizes the importance of the hypnotist's skill and ingenuity in accessing the subject's hypnotic capacities in ways which are unique for each individual.

Although it is possible to practice hypnosis in indirect forms without necessarily subscribing to Erickson's theoretical views, some special views about the nature of hypnosis do happen to be associated with the Ericksonian approach. Some of these will be briefly discussed below in the sections on characteristics and theories of hypnosis, but the interested reader is referred to Erickson's publications for more detailed accounts.

Characteristics of Hypnosis

A constellation of characteristics associated with hypnosis help to define it as a recognizable entity. Yet, while each of these might occur with some frequency, few of them are invariant characteristics.

Redistribution or fixation of attention is a characteristic almost always associated with hypnosis. It refers to the focusing of attention on a circumscribed area in order to reduce sensory input (Hilgard, 1963; Kubie & Margolin, 1944). It is ordinarily accomplished by the hypnotist asking the subject to attend to a restricted range of stimuli, such as a metronome, the hypnotist's voice, or a dot on the wall. *Motivation* to experience trance, *belief* in hypnosis, and *expectation* of trance are considered by researchers to be among the more significant factors helpful in characterizing and accounting for hypnotic behavior (Barber, 1969; Barber, Spanos, & Chaves, 1974; Spanos & Barber, 1974). The likelihood of experiencing hypnosis is reduced when there is either low motivation, distorted beliefs about hypnosis, and negative expectations. *Heightened suggestibility,* or openness to suggestion, or disinclination by the subject to autonomously initiate activities, has long been thought to be a characteristic of hypnosis. However, many practitioners (e.g., Erickson et al., 1976) do not believe that suggestibility plays an important role and empirical research has indicated that increases in suggestibility are not as great as has been commonly assumed (Ruch, Morgan, & Hilgard, 1973).

Hypnotic subjects typically accept some degree of *reality distortion,* showing an ability to accept suggestions which would not ordinarily be accepted, such as for hallucinations. *Trance logic* is another characteristic which may be related to reality distortion. Trance logic permits the subject to register reality at one level while remaining unaware of it at another, resulting in the acceptance of suggestions and situations which would ordinarily be immediately judged as illogical or incompatible with reality considerations (Bowers, 1976; Orne, 1959). However, studies on trance logic have yielded conflicting findings (Hilgard, 1972; Johnson, Maher, & Barber, 1972; Sheehan & Perry, 1976) and have provided little justification for considering trance logic to be an invariant characteristic of hypnosis. It is probably safer to conclude that trance logic occurs only in some subjects and in some trances.

Increased role-taking ability is another characteristic of hypnotic experiences (Sarbin, 1950; Sarbin & Coe, 1972). Adoption of certain role behaviors is facilitated by the permissiveness and expectations associated with the hypnotic context, in which reality testing and conscious restraints on behavior are momentarily put aside. The subject is enabled to adopt the role of a good hypnotic subject, or the role of a person experiencing anesthesia, or the role of him or herself at another point in development in an age regression.

Most theorists and practitioners believe that hypnosis is characterized by an *altered state of consciousness* (Bowers, 1966; Orne, 1959). However, this characteristic is difficult to operationalize and to produce in a uniform manner because the subjective experience during trance varies a great deal among different subjects. Since some subjects do not report unusual subjective experiences and yet are capable of manifesting standard hypnotic responses, the question of whether hypnosis does involve an altered state of consciousness is a matter of debate (Barber, 1969). The answer to this question may depend on how altered state is defined.

Trance depth and *hypnotic susceptibility* are variables commonly used to characterize hypnotic experiences. The assumption is that subjects vary in hypnotic susceptibility and that any trance can be characterized by a given level of depth. Mild levels of depth are associated with a restricted range of hypnotic phenomena, such as relaxation and eye closure, while greater levels of depth are associated with a greater range of more dramatic phenomena, such as amnesia and hallucination. These variables are controversial ones and some workers in the field have rejected them as useless. For example, Wagstaff (1981) has observed that it seemed contradictory that people who could tolerate surgery under hypnosis were not necessarily the same people who were hypnotically susceptible by traditional criteria.

It is also possible that trances are qualitatively rather than quantitatively

different from one another; that is, that there are different types of trance
for different people. This possibility is concealed when trances are viewed
along a single continuum of depth. For example, White (1937) has differentiated between two kinds of trance which are qualitatively different,
active and passive trances, rather than different in terms of depth. Belief
in this latter view does not preclude use of standard "deepening" procedures. These can still be used, not to "deepen" the trance, but rather
to facilitate a particular kind of trance experience.

Theories of Hypnosis

A number of theories have been formulated to attempt to account for
or explain hypnosis, some of which are based on one or more of the
common characteristics described above. Some early conceptions of hypnosis regarded it as a pathological state of hysterical neurosis (Tinterow,
1970), as a mental perversion (Witner, 1897), and as a "nervous sleep."
One of the more recent views, from a psychoanalytic perspective, regards
hypnosis as a state of partial regression, with a loss of adult controls and
an increased access to fantasy and impulsivity (Gill & Brenman, 1959;
1962). Conditioning and learning theories regard hypnosis as a habit
learned by practice and reinforcement, which can be initially induced by
cortical inhibition resulting from monotonous induction monologues
(Edmonston, 1967).

Numerous other theories have also been generated in the past several
decades. Of the more recent theoretical formulations, several will be
discussed which illustrate the theoretical diversity that exists and which
provide a relevant background for the working definition of hypnosis
used throughout this book. These have been derived from dissociation
theories and communication theory, as well as from skeptical positions
which question whether hypnosis really exists at all.

Skeptical views. Views of hypnosis have been differentiated into "credulous" and "skeptical" views (Sutcliffe, 1960; 1961), the credulous
views being those which atttribute something unique to hypnotic trance
and the skeptical views being those which posit that there is no difference
between trance and everyday awake behavior. One skeptical argument
advanced by Barber and his associates (Barber, 1969; Barber, Spanos,
& Chaves, 1974) is that hypnosis, as a special state, has been inferred
on the basis of hypnotic responses that it is assumed to cause; that is, it

is circular reasoning to say that the hypnotic responses indicate the subject has been hypnotized and then to conclude that those responses are caused by hypnosis.

Due to this reasoning and to the research findings which suggest that highly motivated subjects who have not been hypnotized can produce behavior usually regarded as caused by hypnosis, Barber and his colleagues believe that there is no special state of hypnosis. They have suggested that subjects carry out hypnotic behaviors when their attitudes, motivation, and expectations are positive toward the test situation; these factors facilitate a willingness to think and imagine with the suggested themes, enabling an imaginative involvement and a responsiveness to suggestions.

Barber and his colleagues are not alone in discarding "hypnosis" as an explanatory concept. Others (e.g., Hunt, 1979; Sarbin & Coe, 1972; Wagstaff, 1981) use the term only as a descriptive concept, preferring to incorporate hypnotic phenomena within the framework of other social psychological concepts, such as role enactment, compliance behavior, or attribution theory. These skeptical views have been useful in stripping hypnosis of its mystery and revealing some factors that help to account for hypnotic behavior. However, by emphasizing that behavior similar to hypnotic behavior can be voluntarily produced, the skeptical positions ignore an important feature of many trance experiences: that hypnotic behavior is perceived by many hypnotic subjects to be occuring effortlessly, that is, involuntarily. Aside from this problem, the acknowledgement by these skeptical positions that imaginative involvement plays an important role provides an important link to theories which invoke concepts of attentional absorption, fixation of attention, or redistribution of attention.

Attentional theory. A significant theoretical position developed by Shor (1959) explains hypnosis as a function of the redistribution of attention. According to this view, a hypnotic trance consists of a temporary orientation to a small range of preoccupations and a simultaneous fading of the generalized reality orientation into nonfunctional awareness. The generalized reality orientation is the "whole abstract superstructure" of relationships and mental representations existing in the immediate background of awareness, which is used to interpret, support, and integrate everything else in reality. As a theoretical construct, it bears a striking similarity to the construct of "tacit knowledge" in the learning and memory literatures and to the construct of "the unconscious" in Freudian and Ericksonian approaches.

While the generalized reality orientation does function to test reality, it consists of more than this function; it is the inner representation of reality itself, which we all must have within us in order to test reality. In normal consciousness, when special aspects of the generalized reality orientation are the focus of attention, the rest of the reality orientation is usually accessible or in close communication. When this close communication or accessibility is lost, the state of mind can be designated as trance, dreaming, psychotic states, or utter absorption in music, art, literature, drama, fantasy, or other subjects. Dissociation is another way of conceptualizing this communication gap between cognitive structures.

Dissociation theories. Hypnosis has been explained by Erickson and others as a form of dissociation, in which some aspects of cognitive functioning are dissociated from others (Erickson et al., 1976; Hilgard, 1973). According to one dissociation theory (Hilgard, 1973), there is a dissociated "hidden observer" in consciousness which continues to monitor reality considerations despite the distortion of usual perceptions of reality. For example, a subject who has experienced a significant sensation of anesthesia might acknowledge, if pressed to do so, an awareness of pain at some remote level of consciousness. The perception of body parts as distant from oneself, the abandonment of conscious problem solving, and the feeling that behavior is occuring involuntarily and on its own are all examples of dissociation.

Communication theory. The subject's perception of hypnotic behavior occuring on its own is considered by many to be a distinguishing feature of trance. A theoretical viewpoint which accounts for this feature was developed by Haley (1958), based on careful observation of Erickson's therapeutic techniques and on Gregory Bateson's theoretical propositions concerning communication and interaction in relationships. According to this view, the subject is able to experience his responses as involuntary because the hypnotist refuses to allow the subject to believe that the subject is engaging in the response on purpose, or voluntarily. To illustrate this, the hypnotic response of arm levitation can be considered.

If the hypnotist asks for the subject's arm to float upward, and the subject lifts his arm on purpose, the hypnotist can tell the subject not to lift the arm on purpose. The hypnotist's communication to the subject is actually a paradoxical one, consisting of a bi-level, contradictory message: Lift your arm, don't life your arm. That is to say, lift your arm, but don't lift it on purpose. If the subject refuses to lift his arm, the hypnotist can agree that the arm should not be lifted on purpose. Yet, the hypnotist continues to send the message that the arm will lift, or perhaps get heavier before it gets lighter. If it gets heavier, or if it gets lighter, and if in either case the subject indicates by astonishment that he is not the one making this happen, then he is engaging in a genuine hypnotic response. He is neither successfully resisting the suggestion nor voluntarily complying with the suggestion. Voluntary compliance would not be experienced as trance, or as different from usual functioning. Genuine trance behavior of this kind is possible only if the hypnotist prevents the subject from establishing the relationship between himself and the hypnotist as either one of resistance or one of obedience. That is to say, the hypnotist refuses to allow the subject to define the relationship between them as either complementary or symmetrical.

Complementary relationships are those in which each person plays a different role, for example, with one person teaching and the other learning, or one suggesting and the other obediently following suggestions. Symmetrical relationships are those in which each plays the same role, on equal footing, such as in competition or escalating conflicts. By preventing the subject from defining the relationship as either symmetrical or complementary, the subject is forced into engaging in a hypnotic response, such as hallucination, relaxation, or arm levitation. It is a hypnotic response because it also conveys a paradoxical message. The message conveyed by the lifted arm is incongruous with the message conveyed by the astonishment that the arm is lifted. This is an incongruity which distinguishes hypnosis from ordinary behavior. In other words, a hypnotic response requires the subject to do as he is told but to deny that he is the one who is doing it. The behavior of the subject in a trance indicates that the subject is not defining the relationship at all and that control of what sort of relationship it is rests with the hypnotist.

What is Hypnosis?

Haley's view of hypnosis is a provocative supplement to the other theories noted and discussed above. Although additional views exist, the ones noted here are sufficient to suggest the diversity which exists in the literature. Despite differences in focus among the theories, as well as outright disagreements between some of them, each makes a contribution to an understanding of hypnosis. Yet, due to theoretical disagreements, conflicting research findings, and the inability of any single explanation to encompass all relevant findings and observations, it is difficult to fully subscribe to a single theoretical position. Perhaps, as Wagstaff (1981) has argued, there is no single process sufficient to explain all hypnotic phenomena. It might be best to utilize concepts from various theories to account for hypnosis and to guide therapeutic practice. For this reason, terms and concepts from diverse theories are freely used throughout this book, and often without allegiance to the theories from which given concepts are derived.

However, this book cannot be said to be atheoretical either, since certain of my beliefs cannot help but be conveyed by implication as well as by outright explication. This situation can create confusion for readers who have beliefs which contrast with my own. Therefore, I will attempt to articulate my own understanding, or working definition, of hypnosis. By having done so, aspects of this work which reflect this theoretical understanding can be more easily differentiated by the reader from other theoretical views.

A Working Definition of Hypnosis

My view of hypnosis is one in which many facets of the various theories are compatible with one another; its sources are most clearly evident in, but not restricted to, theoretical concepts expressed by Haley (1958), Shor (1959), Erickson, and the skeptical positions, all of which are noted above. However, it is a view in which the number of defining characteristics of hypnosis are reduced to a minimum. While many factors are considered relevant and of interest, such as depotentiation of conscious sets, willingness to cooperate with suggestions, persistent acceptance of reality distortion, and so on, there are only two factors which I believe are essential to a definition of and understanding of trance. They have repeatedly appeared in discussions of hypnosis and have been referred to by various terms.

The perception of behavior as involuntary. One of these factors is the perception by the subject that hypnotic responses are involuntary, that is, that these responses feel as if they are happening on their own without conscious effort. Many theorists have commented on the voluntary-involuntary distinction, with most theorists viewing hypnotic responses as involuntary (e.g., Bower, 1976; Orne, 1966; Haley, 1958). Haley (1958) has observed that hypnotists routinely make requests for both voluntary and involuntary responses, progressing from requests for voluntary responses to requests for involuntary responses, with this progression occuring at middle and late stages of hypnotic interactions as well as early stages.

This can be seen in almost any hypnotic suggestion, for example, "As you count to ten to yourself (a request for a voluntary response), you can become more relaxed (a request for an involuntary response)." The involuntary responses are those which seem to occur on their own or which seem caused by the hypnotist in some way. They are not responses which the subject believes he or she has consciously initiated, because these would be perceived as voluntary. Neither are they conscious attempts to obey the hypnotist's suggestions, because these too would be perceived as voluntary. The trance state can be defined as that moment of shift when the subject begins to follow suggestions involuntarily.

Although it can be argued, as Wagstaff has done (1981), that this view is contrary to the subjective experiences of some subjects and also contrary to pre-induction explanations of hypnosis used by most modern hypnotists, this argument is directed more at the myth that hypnotic trance consists of a robot-like obedience. The perception of responses as involuntary is a much more fragile phenomenon. It can also be argued that hypnotic effects can be produced with voluntary effort by nonhypnotized subjects. I do not disagree with this proposition, but point out in agreement that these subjects have simply not experienced trance if their perceptions are that their responses are voluntary ones. Their responses may be described in other ways, but not as trance experiences.

The illusion or subjective experience of responses occuring on their own is a common characteristic reported by subjects who have concluded that there is something uniquely hypnotic or different about their experience. Even in self hypnosis, there is that shift in belief wherein the subject has tricked him or herself into believing that something is happening on its own, though on another level the subject knows that he or she is responsible for what is happening. One can suggest to oneself, "As I count each breath I take, my arm will gradually float upwards and I will become more and more relaxed," with the full knowledge that counting breaths in itself cannot cause relaxation or arm levitation; yet, despite this knowledge, the suggestion for arm levitation and relaxation has been made, and if one can be sufficiently distracted from conscious efforts to relax or to lift one's arm, as well as be distracted from the dubious cause-effect logic of the suggestion, then the hypnotic responses of arm levitation and relaxation can be experienced as involuntary or as occuring on their own.

For some hypnotists who utilize self hypnosis, this process of deluding or tricking oneself into perceiving a response as involuntary is a self evident and necessary component of the trance experience; that it is self evident also implies that awareness of the trick does not reduce its efficacy. The reference above to distraction as a way to facilitate the perception that responses are involuntary serves to highlight the second factor essential to my understanding of hypnosis.

Distraction. In addition to the perception that behavior is involuntary, one other factor appears to be present in most formulations of hypnosis, and some theorists have considered it sufficient by itself to account for hypnosis. It will be referred to here as distraction of attention, though it has been variously referred to as redistribution of attention, attentional absorption, a fading of the generalized reality orientation, fixation of attention, imaginative involvement, as well as by other descriptive terms. The reason that the term "distraction" is preferred to "redistribution of attention" is that only minimal degrees of this factor are present in a great number of instances. Even further, I do not believe that this factor is necessary for trance to occur, but I consider it important to an understanding of trance because it so often accompanies and facilitates trance, as well as help to shape the particular nature of some trance experiences.

These, then, are the two factors which I think best define trance: the perception that responses are involuntary and some degree of distraction (although the latter is so minimal at times that it hardly qualifies as distraction). To describe trance as no more than a combination of these two factors may appear to result in an unusually modest and mundane account in comparison to other more complicated and exotic accounts. However, the degree of distraction can vary, with this variability dictating very different kinds of experience.

When the trance experience involves only minimal degrees of distraction, it may not be subjectively experienced as trance at all, since much of the subject's attention remains focused on usual everyday objects, concerns, and thoughts which maintain a generalized reality orientation. A moderate degree of distraction may correspond to what are commonly regarded as mild trances, while a thorough redistribution of attention may correspond to very deep trances. This does not imply that mild trances must precede deep trances, as does the construct of trance depth; thorough attentional absorption can sometimes be instantly achieved. Also, during progressive stages of a trance, attention may for one reason or another become focused on usual reality considerations, and to the extent that it does, the degree of attentional absorption is diminished.

Compatibility with other theories. The illusion of behavior as involuntary and attentional distraction can account for, or at least are compatible with, most other accounts of hypnosis. For example, the concept of attentional distraction can help to account for the occurence of trance logic and the use of less sophisticated forms of problem solving during trance. Since only a limited number of things can be attended to at a given point in time, distraction to a number of points of focus serves to reduce remaining attentional capacity available for problem solving and logical operations. More sophisticated logical operations require attention to be focused on a greater number of things at once, while more primitive operations require attention on a fewer number of aspects at once.

If, in hypnosis, most of the subject's attention has been diverted to a particular focus where it is held for a sustained duration, any remaining attentional capacity available for problem solving may have to rely on more primitive logical operations, such as those associated with syncretic, preoperational, and primary process thinking, rather than on formal operational and propositional thinking. These constraints on the complexity of available logical operations may facilitate the acceptance of the dubious logic implied in hypnotic suggestions which assert that by the subject following a certain ritual or paying attention to a particular perception, a hypnotic response will be caused.

When the subject's attention is distracted from these kinds of statements, usual conscious reasoning processes are not used to analyze their validity. This is analogous to the suspension of disbelief in the appreciation of drama, which allows impossible events to be experienced as real. The subject can respond as if they are valid and real; in doing so, the characteristics of heightened suggestibility or persistent acceptance of reality distortion might be attributed to the experience.

When insufficient attentional capacity is available for everyday concerns, the usual restraints on playing unusual roles may not be noticed, resulting in a disinhibiting effect, not unlike the effects of alchoholic intoxication. The result may be observed as an increase in role playing ability. A disinhibiting effect of this kind may also be responsible for the loss of adult controls which psychoanalytic theory explains as a regressive state.

Dissociation can be understood as an extreme absorption of most attentional capacity on a selected facet of experience, with any remaining attentional capacity focused on reality considerations as a ''hidden observer'' (Hilgard, 1973). Various examples of dissociation can also be viewed as perceptions that responses are involuntary. Depotentiation techniques are also aimed at neutralizing, or depotentiating, effortful problem-solving attempts so that novel healing responses can be experienced as occuring on their own. Depotentiation techniques sometimes accomplish this by elegantly and thoroughly absorbing a great deal of attentional capacity with insoluble problems and puzzles.

Concluding Remarks

Other characteristics and theoretical views of hypnosis could also be understood, on a hypothetical and speculative basis, in terms of these factors of attentional distraction and the perception that behavior is involuntary. Admittedly, the comments above have been rather speculative in attempting to seek compatibility among various theoretical formulations. What is important is that a system of conceptual linkages exists or can be created among different theoretical accounts, a system which can be helpful as a working model in devising strategies of approach for clinical practice. In such a system, essential factors can be reduced to a minimum, while relevant and useful concepts from diverse theories remain viable for use as needed.

Other ingredients may be quite relevant at times but are not considered essential in any explanatory sense. Much of what has been considered explanatory in the literature and in general practice is considered here to be no more than the colorful trappings and theoretical baggage which, through historical accident, social myth, and cultural conditioning, we have come to believe are central to an understanding of hypnosis. While trance is considered to involve only the two ingredients discussed, "hypnosis" may be considered to involve all the concepts, myths, theoretical baggage, and motifs associated with the evolution of hypnosis over the past two centuries. Included in the latter are concepts of depotentiation, trance logic, suggestibility, role playing capacity, as well as stereotypes we have of skillful induction, such as use of a low soothing voice, piercing eyes, and so forth. To the degree that importance is attributed by the subject to any of these characteristics, they take on potency and can be deliberately maximized to increase hypnotic effects. However, they are not necessary to induce trance or to effectively apply hypnotic methods.

In addition to the two central and numerous ancillary ingredients that help to explain or describe hypnotic trance, trance also must be understood in terms of the specific methods or set of operations used by the hypnotist to produce it. These include the hypnotist's methods for facilitating rapport, making suggestions, creating confusion, depotentiating conscious sets, distracting attention, and employing hypnotic forms of language. While these methods are well understood in the general practice of hypnosis, they are applied in modified forms in those settings which are not ordinarily considered hypnotic ones. The ways in which some of these hypnotic methods can be applied in nonhypnotic contexts are discussed in detail in the following chapter.

3

GENERAL APPLICATIONS OF HYPNOTIC METHODS IN NONHYPNOTIC THERAPIES

Trance experiences often occur in everyday life, but go unrecognized as hypnotic phenomena. They also occur accidentally and with some frequency in therapeutic settings; when they do, even the therapist may be unaware that the client is experiencing trance. The purpose of the present chapter is to describe how hypnotic methods can be utilized with deliberation in therapeutic settings. The result of this deliberate use of hypnotic methods is often a trance which the client does not expect and of which the client remains unaware.

However, induction of an identifiable trance is not usually important; it is more important to utilize hypnotic methods to accomplish certain therapeutic goals. The occurence of a trance which is easily recognizable as a trance is an incidental, interesting, but unnecessary event. It is useful here for descriptive purposes as a reference point because it illustrates some equivalence between these applications of hypnotic methods and the more commonly known applications in which the purpose is to induce an identifiable trance. Therefore, the application of hypnotic methods will often be illustrated in this chapter as if these methods were being applied for the purpose of inducing trance.

First, a few words will be said concerning why these trances go unrecognized and the equivalence of these trances to common, everyday experiences. The remainder of the chapter is devoted to detailed guidelines for application of hypnotic methods in settings not ordinarily associated with hypnosis.

Everyday Trance

The reason why unexpected trances often go unrecognized is that people are generally unfamiliar with the characteristics of trance. Another explanation provided by Erickson and others is that these trances are rather mild in depth (Erickson et al., 1976; Erickson, 1983). A trance which a person does not expect and of which that person remains unaware must of necessity remain a light one. If the trance involved recognizable and classic hypnotic phenomena associated with "deeper" levels of trance depth, then the person would recognize the experience as hypnotic and the trance could no longer be said to be one of which the person remained unaware. A light trance is sufficient for most therapeutic purposes and has been referred to by Erickson as a "common everyday trance" (Erickson et al., 1976). Its observable characteristics sometimes include a fixation of attention, slowed respiration rate, slowed eyeblink reflex, a reduction in random bodily movements, and a smoothing out of facial features due to relaxation of the musculature.

It is easy to see why this sort of trance has been referred to as an "everyday trance." Our everyday lives are filled with moments in which our attention is so thoroughly absorbed that we are hardly aware of anything else. This means that we are hardly aware of those other aspects of the environment which help to anchor us in a generalized reality orientation. Yet, I find it difficult to view all everyday trances as light in depth. Some are rather deep, judging from characteristics associated with greater trance depths which can sometimes be observed. I think it is more useful to simply say that unfamiliarity with characteristics and definitions of trance can account for the fact that everyday trances go unrecognized as trances.

A few common examples of everyday trance include being "swept away" by a good story or a movie, becoming absorbed in the creation of art or in writing, feeling entranced by an interesting teacher or by stimulating conversation in an ordinary interaction, and becoming wholly involved in a daydream or in the ironing of a shirt. When our attention is absorbed in this way, we sometimes engage in overlearned skills and behaviors or act on implicit knowledge we did not know we possessed in a manner that is distracted enough for us to feel as if what we are doing is involuntary, that is, that it is happening on its own without requiring volition or conscious effort.

For example, when swept away by a good book, we are hardly aware of the effort and skills required in the process of reading; the complicated process of reading seems to occur on its own. The perception or illusion of complicated cognitive processes occuring on their own is also reflected in the comments sometimes made by writers when they describe how a book seemed to ''write itself,'' so much so that they had to practically tear themselves away to eat meals or perform other chores requiring conscious effort. Feeling as if behavior is occuring on its own is not a feeling reserved for special endeavors such as the production of art; it happens a great deal of the time to most of us and it happens because it is impossible to remain consciously aware of all the skills and knowledge we use to accomplish even the most trivial tasks. When we are absorbed in any of these ways, whether it be in the creation of art or the mopping of a floor or the weeding of a garden, it is at times typical for all of us to respond to interuptions from phone calls by speaking in such a way that we are sometimes asked if we have just been awakened from sleep; this is a telling comment because it punctuates the notion that these experiences and trance are essentially equivalent.

The capacity to experience this kind of trance exists in everyone and can be accessed with intent in therapeutic settings. The purpose for doing so is not to produce ''trance'' as such, but rather to facilitate therapeutic change; it is implicitly assumed here that most kinds of therapeutic change, whether in contexts associated with hypnosis or not, are accompanied by trance as trance is defined in previous and subsequent chapters. Since it is usually unnecessary to convince clients that trance or hypnotic efforts have occured in order to bring about therapeutic change, it is then unnecessary to utilize methods which implicitly announce ''Here comes hypnosis.''

Hypnotic methods can usually be employed without the fanfare, the anxiety, or the time-consuming explanations which sometimes accompany formal hypnotic inductions. Formal inductions sometimes put too much pressure on the client, risk the therapist's credibility as a hypnotist if he should fail to induce a formal trance, or draw too much critical attention to the therapeutic suggestions. A formal trance induction sometimes requires explanations about hypnosis which consume more time than the explanations are worth relative to the therapeutic goals. These situations may also involve interactions irrelevant to the therapeutic goals, such as conversations about whether or not the client did indeed experience a trance when only a ''light'' trance was induced.

The deliberate application of hypnotic methods or the occurence of trance in therapeutic contexts not ordinarily associated with hypnosis might very well go unrecognized by an observer who did not know what to look for or who did not know in advance that hypnotic methods were being used. Interwoven into ordinary interaction might be therapist behaviors which reflect attempts to redistribute the client's attention, depotentiate conscious sets, and to apply other hypnotic methods for some therapeutic purpose.

Application of Methods

The specific ways in which various hypnotic methods are applied in nonhypnotic contexts is best made clear in the subsequent chapters which contain illustrations in clinical contexts. In contrast, this chapter avoids case presentations and concentrates on providing descriptions and guidelines for the general application of each method. The ways in which each can be applied are described in terms which are as concrete and mechanical as possible in order to clarify their potential for use in therapeutic situations.

Each description of a method includes a contrast to how that method is employed in more traditional and more direct approaches to hypnosis. The purpose of providing these contrasts is to illustrate the continuity between direct and indirect applications of hypnotic methods and to give some idea of the flexibility with which they can be employed. This may also serve to provide a partial review of how these methods and principles are applied in the general practice of hypnosis.

Redistribution of Attention

Since induction of trance and the efficacy of hypnotic suggestion is often facilitated by redistributing attention and capitalizing on the limits of attentional capacity, a few words will be said here about attentional processes prior to a discussion of how these processes can be manipulated. Attention is a complicated construct with many facets and links to other constructs. Orientation, selective attention, attention span, perception, consciousness, and short term memory are only a few of the notions and constructs that have contributed to an understanding of attentional processes. The aspects of attentional processes which are of interest here are those of selective attention. Attention must be considered to be selective because it is impossible to attend simultaneously to all stimuli which are either internally produced or which impinge on the senses.

This limitation has been of interest to researchers of memory who have found that most people can attend to only about seven chunks of information at a time. For example, one popular model of short term memory (Atkinson & Shiffrin, 1967) conceptualized this limitation as a sort of bin which has a maximum capacity for storing chunks of information. When more than the maximum number are entered, some must be kicked out. This memory phenomenon has also been described by other investigators as a limited capacity retrieval system (Watkins, 1974), as a process of rehearsal of information within the limits of attention (Craik & Lockhart, 1972), as immediate memory, and as working memory. The implication of any of these views is that one can attend to, or be conscious of, only a limited number of chunks of information at a time.

These chunks of information can include thoughts, awareness of feelings, memories, anticipations, and also perceptions of the immediate environment which help to anchor or orient a person to his or her usual view of reality. In the induction of trance, the hypnotist capitalizes on the fact that a generalized reality orientation is maintained by a very limited attentional capacity. The hypnotist attempts to fixate or redistribute the client's attention by distracting attention from those several stimuli on which attention is ordinarily focused and which maintain a generalized reality orientation. When this redistribution of attention is successful, the client may seem to lack awareness of the current context or of other perceptions of which he or she is ordinarily aware, which contributes to the subjective recognition of being "out of it" or in a trance; the client also has less attentional capacity available to challenge the questionable logic of hypnotic suggestions.

In more direct inductions, it is possible to simply and directly ask the client to fix his or her attention on some point of focus, whether it be on the hypnotist's eyes, a spot on a wall, the sound of a metronome, or a swinging pendulum. However, in indirect inductions the therapist often brings about a fixation of attention without directly asking for it. There are numerous ways of accomplishing this. The therapist can shift into a slightly different pattern of speaking, characterized by a lower voice tone, slower rhythm, and different semantic content. The therapist can also move his or her body in slow motion, but not quite slow enough for the client to recognize exactly what it is that is unusual about the situation. A shift of this kind is not great enough to be consciously identified as a noticeable difference but is sufficient to attract and maintain attention. Shifts in body position and eye contact are also especially effective.

For example, the therapist can subtly increase the degree of eye contact with the client. The subtlety with which this is done is important. If the therapist suddenly fixed his eyes on the client and maintained a stare, the client could quickly become uncomfortable and mistrustful. This is a perfect example of poor eye contact rather than good eye contact. When people experience with one another what they consider to be "good eye contact" they nevertheless continue to glance away momentarily, at a predictable rate of occurence. This glancing away is essential to maintaining an optimal degree of comfortable eye contact. To use eye contact to bring about a redistribution of attention, the therapist can maintain eye contact just beyond the point of time at which it would have been comfortable to glance away, and at that later point can glance away. This provides an event which is just unusual or incongruous enough to rivet the client's attention, but not unusual enough for the client to need to consciously organize and interpret exactly what the therapist is doing. The maintenance of eye contact can then be gradually increased, with the rate of increase dependent on the client glancing away at reduced rates of occurence.

Subtle applications of this kind appear rather technical but they can be implemented in a very natural, flowing style, just as can any other therapeutic method. If these methods feel to the therapist as if they are too contrived or manipulative, then they are likely to be applied awkwardly and with manipulative intent and should probably not be used. The therapist can use other methods to accomplish the same purpose which feel more comfortable or more natural. For example, redistribution of attention can also be accomplished in more ordinary ways, by conversation or storytelling or questioning which focuses the client's attention on inner experiences, memories, or other topics unrelated to the current context.

In addition to redistributing attention prior to making therapeutic suggestions, it is useful to maintain a fixation of attention while suggestions are being made, but this does not usually require any special measures which have not already been mentioned. After suggestions have been made, it is sometimes useful to redistribute attention again, but in reverse, focusing it on perceptions which restore and maintain a generalized reality orientation. This can be done by returning to usual topics of conversation and reversing the shifts in speech pattern, body position, or degree of eye contact made earlier, once again behaving and speaking in more usual ways and avoiding discussion of suggestions given during the session.

This reversal is equivalent to "trance termination" in more formal uses of hypnosis. In settings not associated with hypnosis, the therapist may wish to reverse the attentional redistribution either rapidly or gradually, just as in formal trance termination. A gradual redistribution or termination is less likely to result in confusion or disorientation or a perception of having experienced trance. However, at times, the therapist may wish to make rapid shifts in speech, tone, rhythm, and so on, in order to facilitate something akin to a partial amnesia that will protect hypnotic suggestions from interference by the client's usual strategies of conscious scrutiny and analysis. An abrupt shift in the therapist's and client's interaction to a more typical interaction is analogous to an abrupt awakening from sleep, following which it is difficult to remember the details of a dream. The details of dreams or hypnotic suggestions are more likely to be remembered and critically examined during a gradual orientation to everyday reality. This kind of critical examination of suggestions can sometimes be avoided by rapid termination, but the probability also increases that the client will recognize that something like a trance might have occured. When this recognition has been made, it has never constituted a problem in my exprience; because the "trance" is equivalent to everyday experiences, clients tend to feel curious and interested in the fact that hypnotic methods have been used rather than feel tricked.

Depotentiation of Conscious Sets

In order to increase the probability that hypnotic and trance inducing suggestions will be accepted uncritically, it is useful to depotentiate, or disrupt, the clients usual conscious sets of expectation, strategies of thinking, and orientation to the current context. Depotentiation results in the client feeling puzzled, uncertain as to what to do next, and wishing to let go of conscious efforts to figure things out. Therefore, it allows the client's experience to be more easily restructured by suggestions. Some of the techniques described above for fixating attention may sometimes serve the function of depotentiation. Since these techniques depotentiate, or prevent, conscious efforts to change and to make things happen, they also help to foster the perception that hypnotic and therapeutic responses are occuring involuntarily or effortlessly.

An actual inner sensation is experienced by some people when depotentiation occurs. The sensation is probably associated with a sudden and slight variation in arousal level, due to the violation of expectation created by the therapist in the effort to cause the depotentiation. In this way, depotentiation is similar to the experience of wonder, humor, surprise, curiousity, and other responses generated by violations of expectation. When a definite physical sensation is experienced, it can ratify for the client that something unusual is in the process of occuring.

In addition to the methods for fixating attention, there are numerous other ways to depotentiate conscious sets in the process of trance induction. Puzzles, paradoxes, contradictions, and Zen koan's are often effective because they occupy a great deal of conscious attention with temporarily insoluble problems and result in the desire by the client to give up or let go of conscious strategies of problem solving. At times, it is useful to crystallize and exaggerate a client's conflict into a paradox or story that rivets, paralyzes, and thoroughly occupies the client's conscious attention. A client's problem can often be related to a parable, proverb, or story from the therapist's own experience. Other stories which are effective in this way can be found in books of folktales within various ethnic and philosophical traditions.

Another interesting depotentiation technique consists of the manipulation of pauses used during a conversation, monologue, or story. Pauses can be used to build expectations and to then violate these expectations. This manipulation of pauses is illustrated in a transcript in Chapter Seven where it was applied in the recitation of the alphabet. The recitation went as follows.: ". . . . to learn the letter A (pause of two seconds), B (pause of two seconds), C (pause of two seconds), D (pause of two seconds), E (pause of four seconds), F (pause of two seconds) . . . . "

This process depotentiates conscious sets by building an expectation that letters will follow at intervals of roughly two seconds and then violating that expectation by pausing for three or four seconds. When the longer pause occurs, a definite sensation is experienced by some people. The violation of expectation is slightly puzzling and the client is unsure of what to do or of what will occur next. When the therapist next speaks, it is to lead the client with a suggestion. To experience the sensation caused by the violation of expectation, the reader can experiment with him or herself by reciting and manipulating any predictable sequence of things, such as letters, numbers, words of a song, and so on. The process can be applied with even more subtlety in everyday conversation, as well as with predictable sequences, but these applications are more difficult to illustrate briefly and with clarity than are applications involving numbers or letters.

Another effective method for depotentiation is that of thoroughly occupying the client's attention, but with the intent to demonstrate to the
client the limitations of conscious attentional capacity in order that the
client give up and let go of conscious efforts. For example, the therapist
can tell the client that he or she obviously has not been able to solve his
or her own problem by conscious efforts alone, and to explain that the
reason why is that we can be conscious of very little at any given moment.
The client is told that in order to help ourselves, and even in order to
accomplish the most trival everyday tasks such as brushing our teeth or
stepping down from a curb, we must trust in our unconscious or tacit
knowledge, that is, all those processes, thoughts, memories and abilities
of which we cannot be immediately conscious. Then, these ideas can be
demonstrated to the client by a monologue which continually redirects
the client's attention. An example follows below.

"As you sit here, you can be conscious of several things, such as me,
my voice, certain thoughts that are occuring to you right now, perhaps
certain feelings or sensations, perhaps of tenseness or a feeling of comfort,
or an itch, or a sense of warmth. And you may notice in being conscious
of these things how difficult it is, even impossible, to be conscious of
every single one of these things that is happening around you and within
you. You may not be at all conscious of the color of the wall, until I
mentioned it to you just now, or the sensation of your foot as it rests on
the floor, or the feeling of hollow space inside your mouth, or the fact
that one leg might be more relaxed than the other, or the sounds in the
hallway, or the memory of a certain coat hanging in your closet at home,
or any number of other things that you know but are not attending to and
are not immediately conscious of. And in becoming conscious of each
of these things I am mentioning to you, you can notice that you may
have forgotten to be conscious of one or another of them, such as the
color of the wall or a certain thought you had several seconds ago or the
sensation of your foot resting on the floor, because all of us can only
attend to only several things at once, and in fact do not need to remember
and do not need to pay attention to every little thing that we know in
order to accomplish almost anything we do. We can simply let go and
trust in all we know and in all we can do, without needing to try to do
anything at all."

This method challenges the client to try to consciously attend to a great
deal and results in the client realizing that he or she can attend to very
little. The client then gives up in this effort and follows the leading
statements by the therapist. The method capitalizes on, and demonstrates

to the client, the limitations of conscious attention by continually redirecting attention to one focus after another. This and other monologues which continually redirect attention can be unobtrusive methods for keeping conscious attentional processes as occupied as possible. They are similar to techniques in more direct approaches to hypnosis in which the client is asked to count each breath as the therapist continues speaking, or is asked to sort into piles imaginary jelly beans according to color while counting each jelly bean, or to develop an imaginary script in an imaginary love scene. These measures prevent the usual processes of attention and conscious problem solving from critically examining the therapist's suggestions. The client is rendered more receptive, less critical, and less likely to question the very questionable logic contained in hypnotic forms of language usage. Also, because these techniques depotentiate the belief that behavior depends on conscious effort, they help to make therapeutic change feel effortless.

The Perception of Behavior as Involuntary

teristic which gives expected trances a "hypnotic" aura, this illusion is important for a different reason in therapeutic situations which are not ordinarily associated with hypnosis. Rather than trying to get the client to feel as if his eyes are closing on their own or that his arm is levitating, the goal is to help the client to feel that the presenting problem diminishes on its own. This is important because it indicates that significant change has occured and that the client is not engaging in efforts which would maintain the problem. For example, trying to not "want to smoke" can only fail because wanting or not wanting something is an involuntary response. Efforts to not "want" serve only to make one more aware of the want and help to maintain the problem. Therefore, the therapist needs to convey the message that improvement will occur but needs to avoid conveying the message that the client should consciously "snap out of it."

Paradoxical and hypnotic methods elegantly address this dilemma because these methods always convey a bi-level, paradoxical message that the client should change but should not change on purpose. This can be illustrated by the following statements, which in this instance are expressed quite simply rather than subtley. "Stop trying to not want to eat. Feel free to want to eat and to want this as much as you like. Wanting to eat is not within your control. What is within your control are some other things you can do which can help you with this problem."

Although convenient, it is probably inaccurate to refer to the perception that behavior occurs on its own as an illusion; the word illusion implies a false belief. Since we can be immediately conscious of only a few of the multiple external factors and internal cognitive processes which influence our behavior, it might be more appropriate to view as an illusion the belief that behavior is voluntary, rather than the opposite. That is why it is so easy to facilitate the opposite perception that one's behavior is happening on its own. That is, it usually happens on its own anyway.

Therefore, it is not usually difficult to foster the perception that improvement can feel effortless. The therapist simply gives the client something to do, such as sitting and listening to the therapist or engaging in some technique or ritual, and conveys the implicit message that by doing this, improvement will occur. The therapist can also make the direct suggestion that the improvement will occur on its own, or that the client need not try to make it happen, and the therapist can even expand on this by explaining portions of the above discussion.

If the client resists by a symmetrical maneuver, for example, by saying that the problem is not improving or getting worse, the therapist must refuse to respond in a symmetrical fashion and instead utilize the meta-complementary maneuver of agreeing that the problem is still quite bad. This consists of backing away from an ineffective leading suggestion and utilizing statements that pace or mirror the client's experience. If on the other hand the client engages in the complementary behavior of compliantly and consciously attempting to get rid of the symptom, the therapist must tell him to stop trying to do this. Thus, the therapist remains in the position to define the relationship and is thereby able to continue sending the bi-level message that the client should get rid of his problem but not on purpose. Much more will be said to further clarify and elaborate on these comments in the following chapter.

Pacing, Leading, & Distraction

Pacing refers to therapist behaviors which track, reflect back, or mirror the client's current behavior. Leading refers to therapist behaviors which influence the client to engage in new behaviors. Leading is equivalent to making suggestions that hypnotic effects will occur. Although pacing and leading are intertwined processes in the practice of hypnosis, each is a separate process in itself.

Pacing the client's current experience has numerous effects, one of which is that the client feels that the therapist genuinely understands and is in tune with the client's point of view. A form of pacing which is used by many nonhypnotic therapists is commonly known as reflective listening, consisting of reflecting back to the client the feelings and ideas conveyed by the client's statements and behaviors. Reflective listening is so potent as a therapeutic method that it is the primary method used in "client-centered" therapy, and is used to some extent in almost all therapies. It establishes a rapport in the relationship between therapist and client which in itself is conducive to positive change and which may be more significant as an effective ingredient of change than the particular therapeutic techniques used or the particular theories or schools of thought to which the therapist subscribes. Therefore, while pacing is described here as a useful method for circumscribed purposes, its more general positive effects on establishing a supportive and trusting relationship cannot be underestimated.

As in any therapy, reflective listening or pacing is used in hypnosis to establish an interaction in which the client feels the therapist is in tune with him or her. This serves the function of enhancing the influence of leading suggestions. When pacing is well executed in subtle and indirect fashions, the client may see in the therapist's behaviors a kind of mirror image of himself; as a result, it may become unclear whether it is the client who is being paced by the therapist or vice versa (although this confusion is not consciously recognized by the client). Therefore, minor and imperceptible deviations in therapist behavior, intended to lead the client to new behaviors, may be assumed by the client to be a reflection of the client's own behavior. These deviations, because they are so minor, may lead the client to mirror the deviations on the assumption that they are autonomous responses. In these ways, more indirect approaches to induction are characterized by leading statements which are unobtrusive, and even undetectible, and by pacing statements which are sensitive and assiduously applied.

In more direct hypnotic approaches, the differentiation between pacing and leading statements is more evident because these processes are applied in forms such as the following: "As you breathe in and out (pacing), you can begin to notice a feeling of comfort (leading). And with each blink of your eyes (pacing), you can become aware of the effort it takes to keep one's eyes opened (leading)."

In less direct applications, the therapist can make use of reflective listening or utilize subtle forms of nonverbal pacing. The latter include mirroring the client's physical posture and movements, utilizing the same vocal rhythms as the client's and matching one's respiration rate and eyeblink rate to the client's. However, if the therapist mirrors the client in too exact of a fashion, the client is likely to recognize this and to feel as if the therapist's techniques are clumsy and artificial. Pacing behaviors can be used in a flexible way that feels comfortable to both the therapist and the client and yet establishes rapport quite rapidly. Both verbal and nonverbal forms of pacing and leading can be used to gradually bring about in the client a more relaxed and attentive state in which bodily movement is minimal and in which respiration and speech are slowed. Illustrations of the multiple ways this can be done appear in subsequent chapters. Pacing and leading are complementary processes which are used not only at initial stages of a therapy session but at most other points throughout the session.

Redirection of attention, in the forms of confusion and distraction, also plays a role in the processes of pacing and leading. In pacing and leading, many statements are made (some of them pacing statements and some of them leading) which are intended to distract the subject's attention from particular leading statements. The particular leading statements from which attention has been distracted have more opportunity to take hold and to be accepted when they are not being subjected to conscious and critical analysis.

The following monologue illustrates pacing, leading, and distracting in a clinical context. The monologue was addressed to a client's problem of work dissatisfaction, illustrated in Chapter Eleven, and was delivered during a therapy session in which the use of hypnotic methods was not overt. The statements used to distract the client from the leading suggestions usually focused the client on a truism, the internal response to which could be easily predicted and therefore paced. That is why some of the distracting statements are also labeled as pacing statements.

"You feel very puzzled that it is easier to get through the workday, when it used to be so difficult. These mixed feelings about work, both good ones and bad ones, are very puzzling (pacing), and you don't like being so puzzled and would like for it all to make more sense (leading). And you know that you've been able many times in the past to discover solutions to such puzzles when you least expected (distracting and pacing), and even now may be beginning to sense that there is a change in attitude towards work which you will be pleasantly surprised to discover is developing (leading). Attitudes are curious things. You don't just decide to have a certain attitude, for example, your attitude towards me, or towards chocolate ice cream, or towards anything else (distracting). You discover suddenly that you have developed one, or are in the process of developing one (distracting and pacing), and sooner or later, whether it is in an hour or sometime tomorrow or in a few days, you can discover it, and feel pleasantly surprised (leading).''

This illustration and the previous description of pacing, leading, and distraction are intended to isolate these processes and briefly illustrate the ways in which they can be applied in therapies which are not ordinarily thought to be hypnotic. More diverse applications can be found in illustrations in subsequent chapters. Before leaving the topic of pacing, leading, and distraction, these processes will be illustrated once again in the description of an exercise for a nonverbal arm levitation.

This exercise can be rapidly applied in therapy sessions to demonstrate that hypnotic methods are frequently applied without the clients feeling as if they are in deep trances. As a practice exercise, it can be useful to nonhypnotic therapists as well as hypnotic ones because it takes the mystery out of hypnotic methods while simultaneously applying them with good effect. It can also be applied as a first step in a formal trance induction when the subject has been led to expect that a trance proceeds from it. More importantly, it is useful for demonstration purposes because the methods of pacing, leading and distraction can be demonstrated rapidly and with uncommon clarity. The technique is analogous to Erickson's handshake induction in which arm levitation is produced by certain subtle maneuvers during a handshake. Although this induction has been previously described (Erickson et al., 1976), it is difficult for many others to replicate because it requires extraordinary skill to apply all the necessary operations in the short span of time in which a handshake occurs. The arm levitation described below utilizes the same operations but in a gradual and drawn-out fashion, with less pressure on the hypnotist to succeed, and with more probability of success, requiring only ordinary rather than extraordinary skill. Yet it has an equally dramatic effect, and takes only a few seconds longer than the handshake induction.

The first step is for the hypnotist to lift the subject's arm, straighten it, and extend it perpendicular to the body in front of the subject. The hypnotist should support the arm in an obvious manner so that it is apparent to the subject that it is the hypnotist, not the subject, who is supporting the arm. Occasionally, a subject will provide initial support and when this happens, the hypnotist may need to indicate, by providing complete support, that the subject does not need to voluntarily hold up the arm. This must be done because it is necessary for the subject to believe that he or she is not supporting the arm in order to experience the surprised realization later that the arm seems to be floating in the air without the apparent support of either hypnotist or subject. If the subject initially believed he or she was supporting the arm, the subsequent levitation would not be experienced as involuntary or "hypnotic."

The subject's belief that the hypnotist is supporting the arm is then paced by the hypnotist's continued support and manipulation of the arm, which constitute continual messages that the arm is being supported. There are three basic areas that can be used to provide maximal support with a minimum of finger and hand contact. These are the wrist area, the upper arm, and the elbow.

By altering the sites of contact, the hypnotist distracts and confuses the subject regarding which site of contact is being used to actually support the arm. Distraction and confusion is best accomplished by providing many rapid touches, some of them providing actual support, but many providing minimal support. It is also useful, for purposes of confusion, to touch all parts of the arm, to travel back and forth across the length of it, and to vary the nature and strength of the touches to include pokes, strong squeezes, gentle squeezes, full hand support, support with only a finger, and so on. Meanwhile, the subject continues to believe that the arm is supported by the hypnotist because the hypnotist continues to provide ample evidence of this by the obvious sensations administered.

While the distraction is occuring, the hypnotist withdraws support from a particular site of contact and simultaneously produces necessary support at another site of contact. As support is applied at the later site, the support should be less than that applied at the earlier site, but only by an imperceptible degree. This withdrawal of support is a leading or suggestive maneuver and is usually accompanied by a barely detectable reduction in the weight of the arm. However, if and when the slight withdrawals of support are not followed by reductions in weight, the hypnotist must be prepared to instantly provide all the support needed to keep the arm up. The withdrawal can be tried again a few seconds later at another site of contact. When the arm is maintained by a reduced amount of support, the hypnotist repeats the process and withdraws further support.

The processes of leading (withdrawing support), pacing (providing tangible signs of continued support), and distraction (rapid changes in site and nature of contact) are used rapidly, repeatedly, and in various sequences until the arm gradually becomes increasingly lighter. As it does so, the subject eventually perceives that the tangible support provided by the hypnotist is not sufficient to actually support the arm. This perception has a depotentiating effect because the subject does not feel as if he or she is holding the arm up with conscious effort. Since the subject continues to perceive sensations suggesting continued support and, paradoxically, continues to feel an increasing lightness in the arm, the pacing and leading process restructures and directs the client's experience so that the client may allow the arm to continue doing what it obviously has been doing, getting lighter.

The hypnotist can add to these depotentiating effects, even after almost no support is being provided, by continuing to furnish progressively and obviously lighter touches and squeezes, especially towards the wrist and hand area. When ready to completely cease contact, light touches in this area add a flourish to the technique because they make it quite obvious that such contacts could not possibly support the arm.

When the hypnotist finally lets go of the arm, it seems to hang suspended. The subject's experience of the arm "just floating there" ratifies the experience as involuntary and hypnotic. This perception is one of dissociation and may further depotentiate conscious sets, leaving the subject with a feeling of uncertainty and a readiness for further suggestions. If the technique is being used as a preliminary to a formal induction, the hypnotist can proceed with the induction. If the technique has been used as an exercise or an illustration, the hypnotist can simply give the hand a gentle push downwards, indicating by this gesture that the arm can return to normal.

The technique provides a useful exercise for those attempting to better understand and apply methods of pacing, leading, distraction, and depotentiation. The application of these methods becomes tangible in the physical contact between hypnotist and subject. The hypnotist can actually feel "resistance" when the arm retains heaviness or becomes heavier. It is also possible in this exercise to fully appreciate the importance of synchrony between hypnotist and subject. One can also feel in vivid detail the process which facilitates the perception of responses as involuntary. Although pacing, leading, distraction, and depotentiation play the most prominent roles in this technique, motivation, belief, and expectation also make a contribution. In exercises, these latter variables can be manipulated negatively by asking the subject to consciously resist, resulting in more lengthy, difficult, but achievable levitations. Such exercises can help both hypnotists and nonhypnotic therapists to refine their understandings of hypnotic methods and to hone their clinical skills. When a therapist can understand and apply various hypnotic methods on a nonverbal level in this way, the application of hypnotic methods to everyday therapy situations can become not only less exotic, but practically self evident.

Hypnotic Language

The kind of language used by hypnotists during inductions and trance work is often quite different than that used during ordinary conversation. This section focuses on the characteristics of hypnotic language used primarily in indirect rather than direct approaches. These include the uses of ambiguity, grammatical violation, pauses, and various technical forms of language usage. A major characteristic of the language used in indirect hypnosis is the avoidance of the directness and specificity which characterize direct approaches to hypnosis. In direct approaches, the hypnotist might make statements of the following kind: "You will find that by the time I count to five you will not be able to open your eyes," or, "You will find your attitude about this problem changed by the time you open your eyes." The directness and specificity in these statements present challenges that the client may easily resist and defy.

The same messages can be indirectly suggested by using vague ambiguities and truisms: "You *can* find your attitude changing, *sooner or later.*" The italicized words indicate the ambiguity of the suggestion. Words chosen by the therapist need to be vague and ambiguous enough to cover many possibilities of client response, yet be just directive and specific enough to provide broad guidelines for positive change. When positive change is slow in coming, the ambiguity preserves the credibility of the therapist's subsequent statements.

Another characteristic of hypnotic language is grammatical violation. In listening to some trance sessions or examining the transcripts of certain sessions, it often becomes evident that grammatical violations are frequent. Whether they are intended or unintended, they can serve the functions of producing confusion and depotentiating effects. Depotentiation and an internal search for meaning occur when a grammatical violation creates ambiguity in regard to exactly what it is to which a given word or phrase refers.

Ambiguities of this kind can also be created by pauses, which are also characteristic of hypnotic speech. Frequent pauses in midsentence, or sometimes prior to and subsequent to single words, can suggest multiple meanings, can trigger imagery and associational processes, can leave the client wondering how the sentence will be finished, and can depotentiate conscious sets by overloading attentional capacity. Because pauses create so many possible effects, they have been omitted in most of the dialogues and monologues used for illustration in this book in order to avoid numerous detailed explanations of them. Although a minimal degree of pausing is depicted in the illustrations, pauses were much more generous in the actual sessions from which the illustrations were taken.

Some technical forms of language usage which are common in more direct uses of hypnosis can also be applied in indirect approaches. These include the use of causal connectives, time-bound suggestions, yes-sets, implied directives, double binds, presuppositions, as well as other forms (e.g., Erickson et al., 1976). Although the interested reader should examine appropriate sources to acquire mastery of these forms, several of these will be discussed and illustrated so that their applications will be recognizable in the transcripts of subsequent chapters.

Language used by hypnotists is almost always characterized by the frequent occurence of casual connectives. "If" and "then" are causal connectives in the following sentence: "If you concentrate on taking ten deep breaths, then you will feel more relaxed and comfortable." The connectives imply that there is a causal relationship between the two statements in the sentence, suggesting that taking deep breaths causes relaxation. Other connectives of this kind include "as," "while," "when," "and," and so on. They serve to connect an assumed cause to an assumed effect. The connection is between an unquestioned fact (". . . as you listen to my voice . . . ") and a questionable suggestion(" . . . you can notice a feeling of relaxation . . . "). The hope of the hypnotist is that the suggestion will be as uncritically accepted as was the statement of fact.

It should be evident that use of causal connectives to link phrases and sentences results in sentences which reflect the pacing and leading process described earlier, with pacing statements providing the facts or causes and leading statements providing the suggestions or assumed effects. Although examples of typical pacing and leading statements in indirect hypnosis have already been given here, another example is given so that it can be considered in light of the causal implications of its connectives: "As you sit here with me talking about this problem (cause), thoughts may come to you that show you a new side to this problem (effect). And as you listen carefully to a story I'll tell you about a similar problem (cause), you may be surprised to discover a different way of dealing with this problem (effect)." Due to the heavy use of causal connectives, paragraphs and even pages of hypnotic transcripts can sometimes take on the appearance of one long run-on sentence. The reader will recognize this run-on sentence effect in some of the transcripts in subsequent chapters.

Time-bound suggestions can also be used frequently in indirect hypnosis. These are suggestions that something will happen at a certain time, but in indirect suggestion some degree of ambiguity is implied. For example, the therapist may suggest that some positive change will occur " . . . . sooner or later . . . . ", or " . . . . some time within the next week . . . . ", or " . . . . perhaps it will occur in a few minutes, or perhaps some time tomorrow, or perhaps even in a few days, or even a week or month, it is difficult to say, but when it happens you will be struck to discover it has been happening." As noted above, these kinds of suggestions are vague enough to preserve the therapist's credibility when the client behaves unpredictably, and yet specific enough to provide broad guidelines for positive change.

An interesting form of suggestion is the implied directive (Erickson et al., 1976). This directive consists of three parts: a time-bound suggestion ("As soon as you know . . . . "), an implied suggestion to restructure internal processes (" . . . . that your hand is becoming numb . . . . "), and a behavioral response that signals when the restructuring has been completed (" . . . . a finger on your left hand will lift"). This type of directive can be readily applied in therapeutic situations which are not associated with hypnosis, as the following example illustrates: "As soon as you both really understand (a time-bound suggestion) that your attitudes about the fighting between you is changing (an implied suggestion for internal change), you may find yourselves unable to maintain those frowns, and may even be unable to keep back a smile or a laugh (suggestion for a behavioral response), feeling pleased that you can let go of all this conscious effort at trying to solve this problem (and, linked to the behavioral response, a suggestion for an affective response)."

Double binds can also be couched in the everyday language used by a therapist in any kind of therapy session. In formal hypnotic settings, the hypnotist might say to the client: "Would you like to go into a light trance or a medium trance?" This sentence distracts the client from the question of whether she will or can experience trance and binds the client to a choice between a light or medium trance. Whichever choice the client makes, she is likely to accept the suggestion that she will go into trance. In therapy situations which are not usually associated with hypnosis, a therapist might say something like the following; "You can make a big change in this problem, or a little change, or a medium change. There are many kinds of changes." Again, these statements distract the client from the question of whether or not change will occur, a question which could elicit some resistance due to the client's previous unsuccessful efforts to change. The client is forced, instead, to address only the question of what kind of change will occur. The therapist's statements assume, and therefore, suggest, that change will occur. If the client then chooses some degree of desired change, she affirms the assumption that change will occur.

Presupposition is a similar form of suggestion, as is illustrated in the following example: "Are you deeply committed to this change you are making?" Again, the question distracts the client from the question of whether change is occuring, which has been presupposed or assumed, and instead asks about the depth of commitment to the change. Whether the client is deeply committed or not, she is more likely to accept the suggestion that change is occuring than to deny that it is occuring.

Another more subtle example follows: "Do the two of you realize, really realize, that your attitudes towards your fighting have changed?" The sentence does not ask the clients to address the assumption or suggestion of attitudinal change, but only whether they really realize it or not. Therefore, they are more likely to accept the suggestion of change, whether or not they realize they have changed.

These and other forms of language usage have been described in more detail elsewhere and the interested reader is referred to these sources (e.g., Bandler & Grinder, 1975; Erickson et al., 1976; Erickson, 1980). Most of them can be employed in general therapeutic situations not ordinarily associated with hypnosis.

CONCLUDING REMARKS

The chapter has described some of the ways in which methods commonly used in hypnosis can be applied in modified forms in therapeutic situations in general. However, there has been no intention to convey the impression that hypnotic methods should be applied only in the ways illustrated here. The illustrations reflect my own particular experiences and my observations of others. I hope that the chapter has illustrated the flexibility with which hypnotic methods can be applied so that they might be applied by others in contexts and in ways which I cannot begin to anticipate.

I also hope that the attention devoted in this chapter to the technicalities involved in applying hypnotic methods will be helpful to therapists. However, there is a danger that my emphasis on a clear explication of these technicalities may frighten some therapists into believing that successful application requires an impossible mastery of technical perfection. Fortunately, most clients are quite patient with our many errors and are polite enough to overlook and forgive most of them. It is their responses to our therapeutic endeavors which helps to refine our methods over time. As clinicians, we can be grateful to our clients for shaping us into more potent agents for effecting change, where the methods we use and the wording of our sentences conform more and more frequently to our ideals of good technique. Yet, no matter how refined our skills have become, our wording of sentences and applications of techniques can usually be counted on to fall short of perfection. It is useful to recognize our errors in order to refine our skills, but this is a never-ending process which is not a prerequisite to effective therapy.

More important than a recognition of a clumsy hypnotic suggestion and an attempt to refine it is the recognition that the effective ingredients of hypnotic methods are inherent in the establishment of a particular kind of relationship with the client, a relationship that constitutes an optimal interpersonal context for change. The establishment of this interpersonal context is the subject of the following chapter. Rather than showing how hypnotic methods can be borrowed in nonhypnotic therapies, as the present chapter has done, the following chapter shows how most therapy can be regarded as hypnotic.

4

AN INTERPERSONAL CONTEXT FOR CHANGE

Integrations of hypnotic methods within various kinds of therapy are illustrated in subsequent chapters but before proceeding with these, it is important to clarify the nature of these integrations. They are viewed here differently than integrations usually cited in the literature which typically consist of the borrowing of hypnotic methods while doing strategic or other types of therapy or the borrowing of strategic, behavioral, or family therapy concepts while doing hypnotherapy. In agreement with Haley (1963), I think that there is little point in differentiating between hypnotherapy and other therapies when it is possible to recognize the ways in which hypnotic methods happen to be operationalized in other therapies.

The ways in which this has been done throughout history have not usually constituted deliberate attempts to apply hypnotic methods, but it is interesting to contemplate Haley's observation that hypnosis has been closely associated with the inception of major therapeutic approaches. For example, Pavolv's experimentation in his development of conditioning and learning theory included the study of what he considered to be hypnotic behavior. Freud's psychoanalytic methods originally emerged from a hypnotic approach developed by Charcot and Breuer during the hey-day of 19th century hypnosis. Also, Erickson practiced hypnosis for years as he gradually developed a coherent strategic approach to therapy in which formal induction procedures became unnecessary and from which recent family therapy models have been partially derived.

Despite an increasing recognition by therapists of a more unified view of therapy and change, therapy continues to be discussed, with some occasional exceptions, in terms of borrowing from one approach to another rather than in terms of a unified structure of concepts. This chapter articulates a unified model which is derived from an interactional view of trance, from which, in turn, the several strategic approaches to therapy have been partially derived. This model certainly does not constitute the last word on a unified view of therapy and change, but only an intelligible and communicable approach to these topics.

It is possible that this model could be viewed as constituting what Watzlawick et al. (1974) might term a "terrible simplification", failing to take into account the complexity of each of the several approaches from which it is derived. However, it is not intended to supplant or simplify any of these other approaches but instead provides a structure within which each of the others has a place. It affords avenues for the therapist to sensibly move, within the same framework of assumptions, from a consideration of the "pretend" strategies of Madanes' approach (1981) to the strategies for second order change developed by the MRI group (Fisch et al., 1982; Watzlawick et al., 1974) to the paradoxical approach of the Milan group (Palazzoli et al., 1975), as well as to other nonstrategic approaches, without having to shift each time to an entirely different framework of assumptions about change and about therapy.

This is not a model of my own invention but rather an articulation of ideas previously formulated by others. The need for its articulation in the present form arose out of the realization that each of the therapies of which I am acquainted or have practiced, especially the "strategic", are to some extent based upon a common framework of assumptions. This common framework constitutes a particular model or way of viewing therapeutic change. Basically, it consists of the therapeutic doublebind and paradoxical approaches to therapy which were developed by the Bateson project, by Erickson, and by Haley (e.g., Haley, 1958; Haley, 1963; Watzlawick, Beavin, and Jackson, 1967). Although these ideas have been previously articulated, it is necessary to articulate them here in some detail in order to illustrate a sensible integration of hypnotic methods with methods from various other approaches.

Its explication here is intended as a practical guide to therapy, at least for the author, and, if nothing else, will facilitate the reader's understanding of the views taken by the author in the various case illustrations. It is intended as this sort of practical guide rather than as a theory, because as a theory it lacks the complexity and refinements which characterize some of the more recent formulations of theory in the field (e.g., Elkaim, 1985 or Stanton, 1984).

It also utilizes concepts which are currently in the process of refinement in the field, such as the concept of paradox. The logical basis for a paradoxical approach has been challenged recently (e.g., Bopp & Weeks, 1984; Dell, 1981.) Some of these challenges are not incompatible with the essential ideas conveyed here. The reader can keep in mind that the term paradox can be replaced by the idea of "polarity" as Hoffman (1981) has suggested or by the idea that contradiction or polarity is a normative process in the universe, or even that paradox may only exist in the mind of the therapist.

The concept of "paradox" is preferred here because it is more familiar to more readers. It's use also preserves the identification of this model with the therapeutic doublebind formulated by those involved with the Bateson project rather than permitting it to be perceived as an invention of my own. Any deviations from the double bind approach are more probably due to my errors in understanding the concept in my applications of it rather than to any intent to create a theory. The model can best be understood as a guide for the practical application of (and I hope not simply a repetition of) Haley's (1963) view of therapeutic change. It may differ from other strategic approaches only insofar as its focus is on the maintenance of a very particular kind of therapeutic relationship, one that is equivalent to the hypnotic relationship. However, this is not a deviation from the concept of the therapeutic doublebind.

In articulating this model, no effort will be made to use language or concepts specific to any single approach. Instead I will borrow freely from all of them, sometimes explaining the same point in a few ways, so that the coexistence of each of these approaches will be apparent. I am not wedded, then, to my choice of language, but welcome refinement and revision, using this language only to create the broad brushstrokes which I hope will convey my essential meanings.

A Model for Therapeutic Change

The model consists primarily of an interface between two conceptual structures, one of these consisting of a specific view of the therapeutic relationship and the other a specific view of clients and their problems. The model can be most succinctly described by the following propositions. When effective therapy occurs, the therapist usually conveys, either explicitly or implicitly, a paradoxical communication consisting of two incongruous messages: "Change, but don't change." That is to say, "Your problem will go away, but do not try to make it go away on purpose." This paradoxical position has been described by a number of therapists, most clearly by Haley (1958). The client is also viewed here as conveying a paradoxical communication consisting of incongruous messages. He wants to change but he cannot change; or, alternatively, he is producing a problem or a symptom, but is not purposefully producing it. The incongruous messages conveyed by the therapist forms a congruous link or interface with the incongruous messages conveyed by the client, and this link catalyzes therapeutic change.

When the therapist can maintain this difficult paradoxical position *vis a vis* the client's paradoxical position, the client can give up a symmetrical struggle with the problem which serves to maintain the problem and can be guided towards change. The client's response of change, equivalent to a hypnotic response, constitutes a paradoxical communication; that is, he is changing, but not on purpose. The client's paradoxical position, the therapist's, and the specific ways the interface between these paradoxical positions facilitate change are elaborated below, each in turn.

Client Position

Clients are often ambivalent about their problems, not necessarily in some esoteric sense, but in a very mundane, everyday sense. They want to change but can't change. That is to say, they want to lose weight or stop arguing with one another, but resist their own and others' efforts to bring about a change. The very nature of a client's complaint, by virtue of it being a complaint, conveys the message that a problem is being produced which the client cannot control by his own efforts. This state of affairs is generally recognized by most therapeutic approaches; I find it useful to view it as a symmetrical struggle or conflict between the client and the problem because this view implies that change can occur when the client is maneuvered into giving up this struggle. This belief is similar to that espoused by the MRI group, leading to the therapeutic strategies of blocking the client's efforts to get rid of a problem because these efforts have been serving to maintain the problem.

This symmetrical relationship, consisting of the client struggling with a problem, can be viewed more microscopically as consisting of a hierarchical incongruity, that is to say, two overlapping, interlocking, complementary relationships which are incongruous to one another; it can also be microscopically viewed as a circular sequence of one-up and one-downmanship maneuvers in which the problem can be considered a part of a system's homeostasis. I know that these are several mouthfuls of technical terms occuring all at once, but I think they are worth reconsidering after they are better understood by concrete examples or by review of the strategic formulations from which they are derived. The symmetrical relationship, microscopically viewed, can be more clearly perceived when the client's problem is embedded in a sequence of interaction involving at least one other person. This can be illustrated by considering a problem of depression in which a nonsymptomatic wife attempts to cheer up her depressed husband but fails.

On the one hand, the wife occupies a superior or more powerful position as helper in a complementary relationship to her husband, who is in the subordinate position of needing help with an overwhelming problem. Yet, because her efforts are futile against this powerful problem, she simultaneously occupies a subordinate, helpless position in a separate complementary relationship with her husband whose depression is too powerful to overcome. This view of the problem conforms most to Madanes' (1981) ideas but is also in conformance or compatible with the MRI approach and with the Milan approach.

The "game", as Palazzoli et al. would term it, is maintained by a homeostatic tension between (or consisting of) a covert alliance between the husband and the depression against the wife and a coexisting (or alternating) overt alliance between husband and wife against the depression, with the husband's alliance alternating (or remaining ambivalent) and the wife's conflict with the depression remaining constant. If the covert alliance were made overt, the struggle between husband and wife would be declared, disrupting the homeostasis or the "game". To insure its perpetuation, there must be no winner and no loser, each remaining unable to define the relationship; each one-up, yet one-down; each powerful, yet helpless.

These combined views from a few major strategic models would lead a strategic therapist to at least block the wife's attempts to cheer up her husband, but that is not the point intended by this illustration and by this theoretical formulation. The point is that in this interpersonal context the wife is almost inescapably engaged in a paradoxical double bind by virtue of the husband conveying a paradoxical message: I am producing a problem, but I am not producing a problem on purpose, or, alternatively, you can't help me, but I need your help.

These messages are conveyed by the husband's complaint about the problem, on the one hand, and by the problem itself, on the other hand. The complaint conveys something like the following message: I am not producing this problem, at least not doing so on purpose, and need help desperately because I can't control it. This message is incongruous with the message conveyed by the problem itself: I am producing this problem, a very powerful problem which you are helpless to control. The therapy is doomed to failure if the therapist responds to only one level of the message by either finding ways to cheer up the depressed man as the wife does (which would doom the *therapist* to a one-down position of failure), or by demanding that the man "snap out of it" (which would doom the *client* to the own-down position of failure because the client would not have consulted a therapist in the first place if he could have controlled the problem by an act of will).

These incongruous messages are conveyed by clients whether they are embedded in systems of interaction involving two, three, or more clients in a family or whether they are conveyed by a single individual. Since it may be more difficult to perceive these communicational or interactional aspects in the case of an individual, individual problems will be briefly considered so the reader can see that these as well as family problems can be understood according to the same communicational, systemic, and strategic considerations discussed above.

Instead of a wife occupying the incongruous positions of being powerful yet helpless in regard to the problem, cognitive processes and feeling states may occupy these positions. As the MRI group has suggested, there is a part of each individual which encourages him to believe that he should be capable of pulling himself up by his bootstraps to solve his problem. This belief is especially reinforced when the individual concludes that no one else seems to have particular difficulty in overcoming or controlling the problem which currently plagues the individual. This belief in one's ability to overcome one's problem constitutes the one-up position which was occupied by the wife in her attempts to cheer up her depressed husband.

Yet, this position leads to predictable sorts of action, such as trying hard not to think about an obsession, trying to feel less depressed and more cheerful, trying to not want to smoke, or trying not to think about feeling afraid of the panic attack that might ambush one at any moment. These are actions that inevitably fail, putting the individual back in the one-down position of feeling unable to control his problem, and maintaining the same sort of homeostatic tension constituting the "game" earlier described. Parts of the self can be viewed as interacting in the same way as the husband and wife in the previous example.

The reader can now easily see how this individual problem can be described either in terms of a series of one-up and one-downmanship maneuvers (the MRI approach), or in terms of a homeostatic tension between overt and covert coalitions or triangles (the Milan approach), or in terms of a hierarchical incongruity (Madanes' approach). One can, of course, view a conflict with a problem as an ego-dystonic situation from a psychodynamic viewpoint, as a failure to be "centered" in oneself from a gestalt viewpoint, or in a number of other interesting ways. However, in the interest of viewing individual and interpersonal problems in compatible terms, I find it most economical to understand them as a circular sequence of one-up and one-downmanship maneuvers or as incongruous, overlapping, and interlocking complementary relationships. On a broader, or meta-level, this interlocking set of relationships consisting of a circular sequence of interactions constitutes for the client a symmetrical struggle with a problem. The client tries repeatedly to overcome the problem and fails, maintaining a rough equality of power between himself and the problem.

Incidentally, when I speak of a client's problem in individual terms, I do so strictly for the sake of descriptive clarity, especially when I do so in the following sections on the hypnotic relationship. It should be evident from the foregoing explication that this model applies to more than single individuals, since its development is based on consideration and analysis of various systemic views of problems existing between individuals, for example, the wife's futile attempts to help her depressed husband.

I do not wish at this point to speculate on the question of problem formation because the answers to this question are not essential to the model I am outlining. It is possible to accept as useful the various hypotheses suggested by others. For example, as the MRI group proposes, it is possible that problems are formed when certain solutions are applied to normal life difficulties, solutions which then serve to make these difficulties worse; or, as Madanes and others have proposed, it is possible that problems are induced or maintained by hierarchical incongruities which place a symptomatic person in a double-binding paradox. Other explanations which are neither strategic nor systemic also appear to have considerable promise. However, the validity of theories of problem formation are not as important to this model as is a way of viewing the problem as it confronts the therapist which can guide the therapist to effective action.

What appears fairly evident in many cases is that clients confront the therapist with a bi-level or paradoxical message: I am producing a problem, yet I am not producing the problem. It is interesting to note that this paradoxical symptomatic response is presumed by some theoretical approaches to be caused by the individual's involvement in a paradoxical situation, such as hierarchical incongruity. It does not matter to the approach articulated here whether or not a paradoxical situation has induced or maintained a paradoxical symptomatic response; what matters is that it is possible to produce or remove such responses by the therapist taking a paradoxical position in regard to the client and the problem. This is precisely what is done in a very particular kind of therapeutic relationship, the hypnotic one. Although an interactional or communicational description of the hypnotic relationship appears in previous chapters, this relationship is detailed again below in order to be understood in the context of this chapter's content. Repetition may also be useful for some readers because a comprehensive grasp of the full complexity of this view often requires more than a single encounter with it.

The Hypnotic Relationship

The hypnotic relationship is one in which the hypnotist conveys a paradoxical, bi-level message which prevents the hypnotic subject from defining the relationship with the hypnotist as either symmetrical or complementary. The bi-level message is conveyed in the hypnotic suggestion for a hypnotic response to occur. To illustrate, the hypnotist asks for a hypnotic response to occur, for example, that the subject's arm will levitate or float upwards. There are two incongruous messages that are sent in this suggestion, either implicitly or explicitly: Lift your arm, don't life your arm. The first part of the message (lift your arm) conveys to the subject that the hypnotic response will occur, that is, that the arm will lift. The second part (don't lift your arm) conveys the message that the subject is not to lift the arm on purpose, that is, as a conscious or deliberate act of will or volition. The hypnotist holds the subject in a paradoxical dilemma by preventing him from responding to only one level of the message. This can be made more clear by considering what happens when the subject responds with either complementary or symmetrical maneuvers.

On the one hand, if the subject attempts to respond with a symmetrical maneuver of resistance (e.g., the arm isn't lifting), the hypnotist must prevent the subject from defining the relationship as symmetrical in this way because such a definition precludes a hypnotic response. Rather than become engaged in a symmetrical relationship with the subject, in which the hypnotist attempts, competitively, to persuade him that the hypnotic response should occur, the hypnotist can remain in the position of defining the relationship by engaging in a meta-complementary maneuver (e.g., by saying "That's right, your arm won't lift, and it can get even heavier before it gets lighter"). By ostensibly taking a one-down position, the therapist covertly remains one-up as the one who defines the relationship. On a meta-level this means that the hypnotist takes credit for the subject's response, defining the response as hypnotic. On the other hand, if the subject attempts to respond with a complementary maneuver of obedience (e.g., lifting his arm on purpose), the hypnotist must refuse to allow the subject to define the relationship as complementary in this way because the subject would then view the arm lifting as a voluntary, obedient response, rather than as a hypnotic one. A hypnotic response is neither a symmetrical nor a complementary response to the therapist.

By remaining in the position to define the relationship and preventing the subject from doing so, the hypnotist holds the subject in a double bind, a paradox, leaving the subject uncertain of how to appropriately respond, since he cannot respond to only one of the two levels of the incongruous message. The subject resolves this paradox paradoxically. When he responds by lifting his arm and indicating by his surprise that he is not lifting it on purpose, his act of arm lifting and his look of surprise convey a double message back to the hypnotist; "I am lifting my arm" is conveyed by the actual arm lifting, while his look of surprise at the arm lifting conveys the message, "I am not lifting my arm." The latter message indicates that he perceives the arm lifting as an involuntary act, that it is happening on its own, and not by his conscious effort. This perception of behavior as involuntary constitutes the essence of trance.

Thus far only arm levitation has been used to illustrate how the peculiar structure of the hypnotic relationship facilitates a hypnotic response. Not only can arm levitation be facilitated in this way, but also tension, hallucination, glove anesthesia, developmental regression, and a host of other hypnotic phenomena. They can also be reduced by the very same principles with which they were induced. It is crucial here to note than many of the hypnotic responses just mentioned are similar if not identical to problems for which clients sometimes seek therapy.

To further appreciate this equivalence, it is useful to note that, on occasion, an inexperienced hypnotist is able to help a client to produce a hypnotic response, such as hallucination or age regression, only to find that the subject becomes frightened of the experience and appears not to be able to reduce it. If the hypnotist also becomes frightened, due to inexperience, and fails to maintain the peculiar but necessary paradoxical relationship with the subject which influences the production and dimi-nution of hypnotic responses, then the hypnotist may allow the subject to define the relationship. He may do this by responding to the subject with a single, congruent message rather than a bi-level message; that is, he will find himself in the position of the wife attempting to cheer up her depressed husband and failing. It will then be the subject who is pre-venting the hypnotist from defining the relationship, rather than vice versa. It is interesting in this regard to note that the Milan group have described repeatedly how symptoms persist as a function of individuals in a relationship refusing to allow the other to define the relationship. It is this very refusal by the hypnotist which permits him to retain influence on the appearance or disappearance of hypnotic responses and of clinical problems.

To summarize, then, a hypnotic response is a paradoxical response to a paradoxical communication by the hypnotist. "Lift your arm, but don't lift your arm" is met by arm lifting and by a look of surprise or a comment which indicates that it is not the subject who is lifting the arm. In de-scribing the hypnotic relationship and the production of hypnotic re-sponses, we find ourselves looking at a mirror image of the description made earlier of a client's problem as it is presented to the therapist. The interface that can be accomplished between these two communicational structures becomes evident in recognizing the identity between them, that is, the equivalence between a symptom and a hypnotic response.

The Interface

By establishing the kind of hypnotic relationship described above which can facilitate the appearance or disappearance of a hypnotic response, the hypnotist can approach a symptom or problem produced by a client as if it were a previously produced hypnotic response, influencing it to increase or decrease in magnitude, just as he would a hypnotic response. At the point of the hypnotist's entry, he is faced with the same situation as he would be if he had influenced the problem to appear as a hypnotic response. The client presents a bi-level message, each part of which is incongruous with the other: "I am producing a symptom, but I am not producing a symptom." Translated to specific meanings conveyed in daily life, this means "I am producing a symptom which is very powerful, which defies my own and others' best efforts to help; yet I am not producing it on purpose and need help from someone."

The hypnotist makes contact with this position by establishing an interlocking interface with it, which consists of his own bi-level message: "Yes, that's right, you are not producing this symptom, that is, not producing it on purpose, and in fact you may as well stop trying to produce or reduce the symptom because it is outside of your volitional control; but it is also true that you are producing this very powerful symptom, a production which can be either increased or decreased in magnitude and which will ultimately be decreased." This is the establishment of a paradoxical relationship, identical to that which engenders symptoms, rather than either a symmetrical or a complementary relationship. The point of interface consists of the congruity which the therapist establishes between the set of incongruous messages conveyed by the client and the equivalent set of incongruous messages that the therapist conveys in turn. To repeat, a congruity is established between two identical sets of incongruities, a link which can also be likened to the connection between two horseshoe magnets.

I am not wedded to the geometric metaphor of "congruity" and I wish to avoid a reification similar to the reification of the hydraulic metaphor in psychodynamic theory. Therefore, I have interchangeably referred to this "congruity" as, and likened it to, an "interface" between two separate information-processing systems, or to the link between magnets, or to the establishment of a paradoxical relationship. Other metaphors, which have not occured to me, may even more aptly capture the intended meanings. What is important is that this interface or meld between the two systems constitutes the therapist's leverage on a problem.

The Therapeutic Relationship

What is most interesting and useful about this analysis of a hypnotist's peculiar relationship to a client with a problem is that it is not unique to hypnosis. A number of therapists are gradually realizing that most effective therapeutic relationships are equivalent in form to the peculiar

form of the hypnotic relationship, even in therapies which are not identified as hypnotic and in which the therapist may have no familiarity with
"hypnosis" and its trappings. This position is in agreement with Haley's
proposition that most therapy is paradoxical. "Paradoxical interventions"
are only one form of application of this therapeutic stance, an application
which highlights the distinguishing features of this stance in the bold
relief of a caricature. The strategic therapies, more than most others,
have recognized this paradoxical nature of therapy and have capitalized
on it in their orientations and their development of various specific treatment strategies. Only some of these strategies are themselves "paradoxical interventions" as paradox is commonly known, but most of them
reflect the paradoxical stance inherent in the model articulated here.

It is easy to see this equivalence between strategies by examining
several of them, such as "paradoxical prescription of the problem",
"pretending to have the problem", and "redefinition of the problem."
Redefinition entails redefining the problem from that of an involuntary
response to a voluntary one. For example, the depressed husband's problem is redefined as one of irresponsibility rather than depression. This
redefinition serves to block the husband's or the wife's demands that he
feel less depressed and instead asks for voluntary, responsible behavior;
requesting the latter conveys the message that performing these voluntary
behaviors will lead to change.

Asking the husband to "pretend" to be depressed accomplishes exactly
the same functions; it blocks demands on the husband to feel less depressed and requests voluntary pretend behaviors, a request which carries
the implication that change will occur. Paradoxical prescriptions which
request that the husband try to feel depressed also block previous demands
to feel less depressed. Each of these strategies alters the way the depression is regarded by either the husband or the wife; the husband and wife
will have difficulty regarding the depression as they did before and will
interact differently in regard to it. Although these and other strategies
fulfill the same functions, their differences are important as well. It is
as if a fundamental approach takes on kaleidoscopic shifts in form and
appearance in order to establish the most appropriate leverage unique to
each problem.

The numerous strategies developed by the MRI group (Fisch et al.,
1982), the "pretend" strategies of Madanes (1981), the Greek chorus
techniques developed by Papp (1980), or the paradoxical interventions,
family rule and ritual prescriptions, and positive connotation strategies
of the Milan group (Palazzoli et al., 1975), are all strategies which may

be effective in themselves but because they reflect the same fundamental approach they help to jockey the therapist into a particular stance in regard to clients and their problems. That stance, in turn, increases the probability that the specific strategies will be effectively applied. A careful reading of the literature on these strategic approaches will confirm for the reader that the therapeutic stance taken by strategic therapists is more important to them than is generally recognized by those who criticize these therapies for an emphasis on specific strategies for problem resolution. The "razzle dazzle" of some of these strategies distracts from the careful attention usually given to the therapeutic stance.

The differentiation between stance and strategy is a somewhat arbitrary one in the strategic therapies. It is more usefully regarded as a blurred boundary or graduated extension of the therapeutic stance which may help to locate the peculiar emphasis of each approach at a particular point than to identify each approach as distinct from others. For example, the focus of Madanes' strategies for marital and for children's problems may appear to readers to be more on the specific strategies themselves as they relate to the presenting problem than on the therapeutic stance, while the focus of the Milan group's strategies may appear to be more on therapeutic stance in regard to the client's paradoxical stance. The focus of the model articulated here is on the therapeutic stance and the relationship between therapist and client because it helps to account for change in hypnotic, strategic, and other therapies as well, enabling a flexible use of various approaches without requiring that their unique values and identities be reduced in order to fit into the present model.

Admittedly, there are some therapeutic relationships which do not conform to the peculiar, very specific set of structures and interactional sequences that have been identified here as the hypnotic relationship. This conformity is unnecessary in a certain class of cases. For example, it is unnecessary in those cases in which the therapist has identified some action a client is taking to solve his problem which serves to perpetuate the problem, advises the client to cease taking this action, the client obeys the advice, and the problem ceases. Other examples consist of a therapist's endeavors to educate or train clients, pointing out errors or providing information of which the client was unaware, with the result that the client uses the information to make changes in behavior which then reduce problems. Therapeutic relationships of this kind are clearly complementary ones, with the therapist giving advice and the client following it. A relationship equivalent to the hypnotic one is not necessary when a direct suggestion for specific acts is followed and results in a diminution of the problem.

However, these are not typical of most cases with which therapists must contend. In most cases, clients continue to struggle with problems even when the therapist gives good suggestions for change. Sometimes clients resist suggestions, engaging the therapist in symmetrical struggles and sometimes they obediently follow suggestions, but do not get better. These are the cases familiar to every therapist, constituting the majority of cases presented for therapy. In each of these, the client has already tried to solve his problem and cannot, remaining involved in an intimate symmetrical relationship which he cannot abandon. In each, a paradoxical message is sent: "I am producing a problem, yet I am not producing it;" or, alternatively, in the form of a request and a dare, "Please help me to change, I dare you to try," or "Change me, but don't change me."

An old Jewish story illustrates a therapeutic approach to this client position. A doctor said to his patient: My friend, you and your illness and myself are three. If you take the side of your illness against me, the two of you will easily overcome me. But if you take my side, the two of us have a chance of overcoming your illness, which is only one.

On the one hand, this story illustrates the client position described here. Yet it is an oversimplification of a complex issue and implies that clients with difficult or resistant problems are deliberately trying to frustrate and defeat the therapist. In contrast to this view, I believe that most clients are desperate for help by the time they make an appointment for therapy, despite giving an appearance of attempting to defeat the therapist at every step. Their degree of desperation may vary in proportion to their ability to defeat both themselves and the therapist because it contributes to the maintenance of the problem. The therapist can respect and capitalize on this motivation and establish influence on the problem by making contact with the client and the problem in a very specific way, a way that is equivalent to the establishment and maintenance of a hypnotic relationship.

It was noted above that there are some therapeutic relationships which do not conform to the peculiar structure of the hypnotic one. The minority of cases for which this conformity is unnecessary has been identified. Aside from this minority of cases, the failure of a therapeutic relationship to conform to the form of a hypnotic one can contribute to therapeutic errors and failures. Examples are numerous and fall into two categories: those therapeutic relationships which the therapist allows the client to define as symmetrical and those which the therapist allows the client to define as complementary. The symmetrical relationships are those in which the client and therapist compete with one another. Obvious forms can be found in the many examples of resistance in the literature and in everyday practice, especially when the therapist views these client behaviors as deliberate resistance and exerts equal or escalating force against it. More subtle forms are also commonplace, but are less apparent. For example, a client inquiring about a therapist's qualifications and the therapist defending himself with great valor in order to persuade the client that he is indeed qualified; or, a client repeatedly responding to therapeutic suggestions with "Yes, but . . . . " and the therapist repeatedly attempting to persuade the client to see the light.

Complementary relationships are those in which the therapist gives advice and the client obediently attempts to follow it. These relationships sabotage treatment when the therapist has advised the client to try not to do something that involves a deliberate alteration of the problem, for example, to try to not think about food in the case of a weight control problem or to try to be more polite and to argue less in the case of spousal conflict. The clients have already attempted various disguised forms of these solutions and would not be in therapy if these had been effective. Advice of this kind, often camouflaged as novel to both therapist and client, fails to take cognizance of the symmetrical struggle in which the client is engaged with the problem and may even exacerbate it. Advice of this kind, with an appearance of many wise and profound forms, is equivalent to the advice "Snap out of it."

Occasionally this kind of "snap out of it" approach does have influence on diminishing a problem. However, I suspect that these instances fall into a special class in which the therapist's physical presence in sessions and psychological presence outside of sessions punctuate for the client that an upper limit has been reached in the symmetrical escalation of conflict between two clients or between client and problem. The alliance of the therapist with the client in these cases enables the client to feel empowered, or more powerful than before, in regard to the problem, or, alternatively, to feel less need to struggle with the problem and able to surrender to it, in either case altering the struggle with the problem in a significant way. This is illustrated by the Jewish doctor's advice in the story told earlier. I am not aware of any characteristics which would predict when this approach, which consists of a congruent exhortation to change, is likely to be effective.

The Hypnotic Relationship Operationalized as a General Therapeutic Relationship

It should be evident by now that what is identified here as a hypnotic relationship is not restricted to a special form of therapy in which the client's eyes remain closed while listening to suggestions, but is rather the very kind of therapeutic relationship which most therapists strive to achieve without being explicitly aware of its parameters. How this approach is operationalized in therapy may require some further elaboration (at the risk of repetition for those who do not require elaboration). Like the hypnotist, the therapist sends a bi-level message which puts the client in a dilemma, preventing the client from responding to one level of the message and thereby preventing the client from defining the relationship as either symmetrical or complementary.

On one level, the therapist sends the message that the problem will be controlled or that change will occur, whether the problem is temper tantrums in a child or depression or headaches in an adult or conflict between spouses. This message is conveyed either explicitly or implicitly, by either words, tone of voice, gesture, implication, or by the very act of the therapist continuing to set appointments and collect fees (even when there is no apparent improvement). The therapist avoids a symmetrical relationship by refusing to respond competitively to resistance or one-upmanship maneuvers; for example, if the client responds to the therapist's implicit message to "Change" by saying that his problem is very difficult and that he doubts the therapist can help him, the therapist can respond by saying that the client may very well be right.

This latter response is incongruous with the message that change will occur and is equivalent to the second message conveyed by the therapist: "Don't change, or, do not try to change or control this problem, but rather give up your futile struggling with it." By conveying the other message, the therapist avoids a complementary relationship in which the client might attempt to engage in the obedient response of trying to control the problem. The therapist prevents the client from interpreting his remarks as requiring this kind of complementary, obedient response. This forces the client to give up his efforts of *trying* to change. In giving up the struggle with the problem, he leaves the struggle behind; for the client, this constitutes a meta-complementary maneuver of surrender which puts the client in the powerful position of defining his relationship to the problem. The relationship is now redefined from a symmetrical relationship of conflict to one in which the conflict has been left behind. This is reminiscent of Jesus' response to the temptation of Satan: get thee behind me.

The allusion to the Jesus-Satan relationship illustrates the point that it is not as important to annihilate a problem as it is to redefine its relationship to oneself. When one struggles with and is in conflict with the temptation to smoke cigarettes, one constantly defines oneself as a person who has just given in to the urge or as a person who has just resisted the urge; or, when struggling to be more polite to a spouse, one defines oneself at each moment as polite or rude. To be or not to be, to smoke or not to smoke, to be more or less polite, all constitute questions which the person struggling with a problem has defined as the crucial ones, and by that definition has created an illusion of alternatives, an endless game, which offers no route for escape or for satisfactory resolution. Definition of oneself in these terms depends on the commision or omission of the problem, its presence or absence. It is this self definition that gives a problem its symmetrical power to persist, a power equal to oneself. When one gives up struggling, it may be that one gives up an inflated view of one's self importance and power, perhaps only the self important belief that one is asking the right questions. That is, one can now take an outside or meta-position of questioning the very question. The result of this surrender is sometimes a more humble view of oneself and an altered view of reality, an altered view which consists of a change in the relationship to the problem: to smoke or not to smoke is no longer a question.

The Equivalence of Trance, Altered View, Second Order Change, and Unconscious Behavior

Describing the change noted above as an alteration in one's view of reality is not just an overdramatic statement intended to emphasize a point. The alteration in viewing reality consists of the redefinition of one's relationship to the problem, that is, redefining a symmetrical relationship of conflict to one that is not conflictual. When struggle with a problem no longer exists, change feels involuntary or effortless. Therefore, the alteration in one's view of reality can be said to also consist of the perception of one's behavior as involuntary, that is, that one's responses of change do not require conscious effort.

This perception by the client occurs when the therapist conveys the message that change will occur (and attempts to engineer such change) and yet prevents the client from engaging in conscious efforts to change which would maintain the problem. When the therapist fails to prevent the client from these efforts to change, the resulting behaviors, even when they have the outward appearance of improvement, constitute what Watzlawick et al. (1974) have defined as first order change (referring to the notions of "more of the same" or "the more things change, the more they stay the same"). This failure can be described as one in which the therapist allows the client to define his relationship to the therapist as a complementary one. If the therapist is successful at preventing the client from engaging in a complementary, obedient response for trying to change, and yet has provided means by which change can occur, then a second order change is possible. If the client were to comment on this change, he would indicate that he could see that he is certainly producing the change but that it is not being produced with conscious effort. The client's paradoxical communication (i.e., changing as he was told to do but denying that he is doing it deliberately) is the same as trance or hypnotic behavior. Trance, then, can be viewed as one type of second order change.

It bears on this point to note that Watzlawick et al. (1974), in describing the difference between first and second order change, indicated that changes in dreams occuring during sleep are examples of first order change but that awakening from sleep constitutes a second order change. The change from a belief that everyday interaction and behavior is consciously controlled to a belief that things are happening effortlessly or involuntarily is a change that can be regarded exactly in this way. This is not to say that a person wakes up or falls asleep when this type of change occurs; that is, I am not invoking the concept of hypnosis as an "altered state of consciousness" akin to sleep, mystical revelations, or drug experiences. It is, instead, to invoke the voluntary-involuntary distinction regarding our perceptions of behavior. The alteration in consciousness consists only in an alteration in perception about whether behavior is voluntary.

Therapeutic changes associated with improved individual and family functioning are not the only ones that occur most efficiently when they seem to occur effortlessly and on their own. Intellectual discovery also feels to the discoverer as if it was not volitional, occuring as if by accident or by god-given revelation, whether this involves scientific and philosophical breakthroughs, solutions to puzzles, punchlines of jokes, or the more frequent trivial insights that illuminate and often guide our everyday lives.

Therefore, when referring to the illusion, perception, or belief of behavior as involuntary, I am not implying that clients, when they change, become automatons. As was pointed out in the previous chapter, this illusion or perception is quite fragile and can be easily shattered and reversed by a successful symmetrical maneuver by the client if the result should prove distasteful or unhealthy to the client. It is a fragile illusion because in our everyday life we tend to view some of our behaviors as involuntary and some as voluntary but often mislabel these and end up rather ignorant and confused about which are which. As a result, we often flatter ourselves (perhaps because it allows us to feel less uncertain and anxious about the uncertainties of the powerful, incomprehensible, and unpredictable world in which we live) into believing that much more is within our understanding and under our volitional control than actually is the case.

Due to the severe limitation on the number of perceptions, thoughts, or bits of information to which we can attend at any single point in time, it is impossible for us to act with conscious deliberation in more than a token few of the many daily acts of eating breakfast, walking up a curb, putting the words of a sentence into a very particular sequence as we rapidly speak to one another, putting our left arm always first (or is it the right?) into the sleeve of a shirt every time we put a shirt on, and so on. Almost everything we might do can be done, and usually is done, without deliberate and conscious attempts to "will" it to occur.

Yet we occupy a precious bit of limited attentional capacity with the reminder that we "must decide on" or "try to do" such and such, as if the completion of a sentence depended on a conscious choice of the sequential arrangement of each and every word in relation to every other, or the stepping up on a curb depended on firing off a string of separate commands to every muscle group involved in that highly complex arrangement of physical processes and actions. These get done whether or not we believe that they depend at every step on our volition, conscious choice, or deliberate intent. In fact if we had to depend on a conscious decision to identify and trigger the *very* first and then the *very* second specific behaviors involved in that complex action in order to trigger the action, we would instantly paralyze ourselves and be unable to even step up on a curb.

Perhaps we are led to believe that our actions depend on volition partly because new learning often requires conscious deliberation and effortful practice (e.g., deciding whether to shift gears before or after turning on the ignition in learning to drive a car) before these actions can be unconsciously and effortlessly performed. Once they can be unconsciously performed, it becomes difficult to consciously identify discrete segments within the sequence of action, and attempts to do so can interfere with efficient performance. The word "unconscious" is used here as an adverb rather than a noun; it is used deliberately to point out some of what Erickson and some cognitive theorists have meant by the term "unconscious," rather than the more Freudian meanings which the word suggests.

I leave the more mysterious workings and rules of "the unconscious" to those who seriously research and study them in cognitive, linguistic, and psychodynamic fields, and to those who personally knew Erickson and who have spent considerable time and analysis on his views of unconscious phenomena. The point that I wish to make here, one which Erickson shared, is that a major task of therapy is to access, utilize, and trigger unconscious action, action that can occur effortlessly; and that this is done by distracting a client from, or depotentiating, the belief that change depends on conscious efforts to will it to occur. To appreciate the importance of this, one must not underestimate how ubiquitous is this belief in daily life that most of our actions depend on volition, deciding things, and "trying"; and one must also appreciate the gratifications and expenses occasioned by adopting this belief.

Reminding ourselves that we "must now try" to do such and such validates for us our belief in our power to control our lives, to be one-up, to have some self importance, even when this reminder is unnecessary to, and perhaps a hindrance to, effective action. That validation then serves to reinforce and maintain the self reminding cognitions. This constitutes a self deception with some interesting consequences. The self reminder requires or occupies a precious bit of our limited attentional capacity (i.e., even if it is one bit, it is precious), and thereby may render us less intelligent, less capable of utilizing logical operations that require attention to a greater number of features at a single point in time. Also, this reminder that one must be one-up renders us vulnerable to any slights to that illusory one-up position, whether these slights are conveyed by others or by our own failings, tempting us to instantly countermaneuver, in valiant struggles, to better control and conquer a windmill or a straw man. As can be seen, the gratifications of this one-up position has its costs; it is a position which is taken at the expense of a more accurate perception, perpetuating self deception and a denial (or distortion) of one's view of the certainties and uncertainties of the world.

These observations on, and implications of, the number of things one can attend to at a given point in time help to account for a confusing phenomenon experienced by everyone: that having arrived at some peculiar insight or point of view or resolve that one believes will help guide one to better living, one finds the next day or the next hour that this preferred view has somehow vanished (e.g., a cheerful view of life or a resolve to no longer smoke or a belief that there is no longer any need to argue with one's husband). One's priorities and beliefs now appear, as if a subtle kaleidoscopic shift has occured, in a new, peculiar, yet familiar arrangement. Feeling confused about this and needing to feel more certain or one-up, we struggle to preserve or recapture the old arrangement, but in doing so we ignore an important fact: that there have been repeated changes in our "viewpoint", that is, repeated changes in the arrangments of things to which we attended at the millions of points of time between then and now.

This is equivalent to the Zen notion that the self is reborn at each moment rather than the self having continuity. This notion was also eloquently expressed by Don Quixote in Cervantes' novel when asked by a neighbor how he could think he was the knight Don Quixote when all knew that he was Senior Quixana, a humble gentleman farmer; Don Quixote replied simply that he knew who he was and who he could be. This is no different than the belief expressed by the indian sorceror Don Juan (Castaneda, 1972) that one can, in an instant, correct, transform, or distort oneself. It helps us to see how sudden change, for the better or worse, can occur without us having to identify a multitude of factors which outline the evolution of a change, factors which we usually seek to provide us with some self satisfaction about our grasp on the world.

The discontinuities in our experiences of who we are, which has just been described above, does not imply that we are entirely different from one moment to the next. What is different from one moment to the next are our objects of attention. If we insist in our theories that we can each observe our "self" or our "ego", then we make this self an object of attention; as such it becomes vulnerable to an infinite number of descriptions and to rebirth at every moment, defying our philosophical and scientific attempts to understand and describe it as an invariant entity. It may be that the part of each of us that observes the objects of attention can not really be observed at all. Therefore, it eludes our best efforts to describe it. Rather than continue futile attempts to do so, it may be more fruitful to find ways to enhance (not to observe) the observing function within ourselves. Several forms of "mysticism" have for centuries been devoted to this goal; the relevance of this goal to psychotherapy has recently been described with clarity and coherence by Deikman (1982). As long as we continue to confuse our identities with the objects of our attention, we can count on having difficulty in keeping track of who we are and in being bitterly disappointed when an illuminating resolve suddenly vanishes as if for no reason.

These observations on our changing "viewpoints" from one moment to the next also helps one to understand why a single therapeutic intervention, consisting of a powerful set of paradoxical demands (Change, but don't change) may be insufficient to produce change. These suggestions would be enough to effect change if one could guarantee that the person would comply with them or remember them all of the time. However, it can more easily be guaranteed that the person will not comply a good deal of the time, not because he is resisting the suggestions but because he does not recognize all of the appropriate moments to apply them. Due to human limitations on the number of things one can attend to at a single moment, he may forget to apply the suggestions, may be distracted from them, or may find that the injunction to comply has less priority at a later moment than it had at an earlier one.

Therefore, it is useful to bind a person in additional ways which preserve the therapeutic message (to cease trying to change) from the vagaries and picaresque wanderings of human distractibility. When the message to stop trying to change is conveyed simultaneously by multiple forms of intervention, a communicational resonance is established which has greater probability of blocking unpredictable ways in which a person might continue his trying to change at any one of the millions of points of time occuring in a day. This communicational resonance can be likened to locking a horse in place by lassoing it from several points at once.

In nontherapeutic contexts where this kind of resonant blocking is not deliberately established, we can pretty much count on the fact that despite our good resolves, things might suddenly change for the worse, and, despite how bad things look, that they can also suddenly change for the better if we would just let it happen. But often we struggle in vain, with conscious intent, to recapture a preferred view and fail, the failure then tempting us to condemn the preferred view as an invalid illusion, and leaving us confused about the continuity of our identities, about who we are.

The only continuity to which we believe we can still cling, then, in our effort to keep track of who we are, consists of the reminder that we must do something or "try" (often a reminder in the form of: "I'm the kind of person who . . . . "), a reminder that perpetuates an illusion that there is a continuity of self, but a one-up self that is never quite one-up enough for reasons elusive to that one-up position, a position which perpetually pursues those reasons. This circular sequence of one-up and one-downmanship maneuvers is the same as the feedback loop described by Bateson in which the organism's discomfort (which is a one-down position) activates a behavior (a one-up maneuver) which preceded the discomfort in a repetitive circular sequence. The purpose is to verify (or challenge) that it is that behavior which brings about the discomfort, a verification which can be achieved when the discomfort reaches some threshold level, sometimes only achieved ". . . . on the other side of death" (Bateson, 1972, pp. 327-328).

Even when this one-upmanship is not intended to control others, it can be viewed at least as an effort to control or define our relationships to others and to things, as has been elaborated more fully by Palazzoli et al. (1975) They liken it to "hubris" or pride, a common human characteristic which in one form or another has been depicted in glorified and tragic forms in the literature, myth, and science of our species throughout its history. Going back even to the beginning of that history, we find that the "fall" from grace by Adam and Eve was due to their self deceptive pride in what they believed they were capable of knowing about the world by eating of the "tree of knowledge." The relationship between pride and our ignorance of the world (or the limitations on what we can consciously know), was aptly captured by Shakespeare when he likened the human to an angry ape:

. . . . man, proud man!
Dressed in his little brief authority, -
Most ignorant of what he's most assured,
His glassy essence, - like an angry ape,
Plays such fantastic tricks before high heaven
As make the angels weep; who, with our spleens,
Would all themselves laugh mortal.
(Measure for Measure, Act II, Scene II)

When one stops reminding oneself to "try", one can attend to one more piece of information than one could before. This incremental change in the amount to which one can attend may appear small but it may render accessible an array of vistas, perspectives, and logical operations of greater complexity, resulting in what feels or appears like a quantum leap, a qualitative or discontinuous change rather than an incremental one; the same perception of discontinuous or qualitative change occurs in reverse when the amount to which we can attend at a given point is markedly reduced, for example, from the effects on attentional capacity of certain drugs, anxiety, brain damage, retardation, and distraction.

In addition to the possible cognitive advantages of surrendering the need to "try" to accomplish most of our everyday accomplishments, there are some other interesting advantages. When one stops reminding oneself to "try" to do this or that, and accepts the humbling fact that things get done without one's willing it (and often more efficiently without the interference of conscious bumbling), one can notice, from a one-down position (even if this noticing should occupy some attentional capacity), that one's behavior is often effortless trance behavior; that is, one is producing it but one is not producing it on purpose. The implication is that the less one "tries" or reminds oneself that acts are volitional, the more things seem to get done effortlessly as in a trance. This is perhaps one of the multiple meanings conveyed by a cryptic Taoist passage in the *Lau Tsu*.

In the pursuit of learning one knows more every day.
In the pursuit of the way one does less every day.
One does less and less until one does nothing at all.
And when one does nothing at all,
There is nothing left undone.

                                        (Book II, Verse 48, Line 108)

In view of these various considerations, it should by this point be quite clear that, since trance behavior is a second order change which is brought about through the establishment of a relationship of the hypnotic form, the relationship can be said to constitute, itself, second order change. At the very moment such a relationship is established, verifiable by the client's paradoxical response to the therapist's paradoxical communications, change has begun to occur and reality is viewed differently. This sounds rather dramatic, as if I had gotten carried away into believing that every client who changes or who is involved in a therapeutic relationship also experiences a vivid moment of entranced wonder and illumination in the noticing of change.

Although this sometimes aptly describes the client's experience, it just as often happens that a little boy who has been helped to make immense changes can barely remember (or, if remembering, minimizes) the distress he experienced at the outset of therapy. This example punctuates the fact that trance, altered view of reality, second order change, and the occurrence of unconscious behavior do not depend on their recognition in order to occur. This recognition is important only if it is important for some reason that the client recognize that "hypnosis" or trance has occured.

Many hypnotic techniques are devoted to facilitating this recognition, but it is usually unnecessary for therapeutic change to occur.

Concluding Remarks

The therapeutic relationship described here can be established in almost any therapeutic setting regardless of the particular brand of therapy being used. While methods of a particular therapy may have curative effects not predicted by the present model, many of these methods do serve hypnotic functions despite the fact that they were not invented for that purpose. For example, "free association," the very foundation of Freud's psychoanalytic method, may have curative functions unrelated to the present model. Yet, his instructions for free association were for the client to observe the contents of consciousness as if observing the passing scenery from the window of a train. This basic instruction is contained in many hypnotic techniques which aim at facilitating the perception that responses are involuntary and that change can occur without conscious struggle. The fact that this and many other therapy methods fulfill certain hypnotic functions is obscured from notice by the stereotyped and constraining conceptions of hypnosis that have dominated the field of therapy until recently. The several ways in which various therapy methods fulfill hypnotic functions will be identified in the following chapter. This will clarify the integration of approaches appearing in the case illustrations of subsequent chapters.

5

THE FOUR FUNCTIONS OF THERAPY METHODS WITHIN THE MODEL

Clearly, therapists do something more than establish a particular kind of relationship and this something more consists of methods or approaches taught by various forms of therapy, such as positive connotation, systematic desensitization, hypnotic ritual, free association, analysis of genograms, mutual storytelling, jamming rigid sequences of circular interaction, reflective listening, cognitive restructuring, and so on. It is important to consider how these methods, whatever they are, might fit into the approach that has been described here. Some of these methods facilitate the operative functions, or effective ingredients, of the approach, while others may serve other functions. Four functions fulfilled by various methods can be differentiated: 1) conveying the message that change should not occur with conscious effort, or blocking client efforts to change in this way; 2) conveying the message or fostering the belief that change will in fact occur; 3) enhancing the probability of change by utilizing potential change agents extraneous to the model; and 4) distracting the client's attention from therapist maneuvers to effect change, maneuvers which fall into the three above categories. These four functions will each be clarified in turn.

Blocking Efforts to Change

The first of these functions is fulfilled by all of the strategies developed by the MRI group; these strategies were specifically designed to block clients from engaging in problem-maintaining solutions. Most of Madanes' methods were also designed to prevent clients from engaging in previously futile helping behaviors. Many hypnotic techniques, such as "depotentiation of conscious sets," serve the function of helping clients to "give up" conscious efforts and to "let go of" struggling. The use of ritual in a variety of therapies also serves to distract clients from futile solutions for change.

Distracting clients from conscious efforts to change is accomplished by many of the methods derived from nonstrategic therapies. For example, the psychodynamic method of implosion and the behavioral method of flooding are similar to paradoxical interventions in this way. They require the client to *have* the problem rather than avoid it. These interventions artfully block the client from avoiding the feared stimulus by requiring that he repeatedly expose himself to it.

Analytic, self-actualizing, and extended family systems approaches sometimes inadvertently block the client's fruitless struggles with the problem by stressing the importance of insight and understanding rather than problem resolution as a prerequisite to change. When done with craft and deliberation, conveying the message that there are prerequisites to change can put an abrupt end to active efforts by the client to bring about an immediate change and focus energy on establishing the prerequisites; once these have been established, the client may be changed in such a way that a problem no longer exists for the client because he negotiates with reality differently. Examples of such prerequisites range from body-building and learning manners to differentiation of the self in one's family of origin.

The function of blocking clients from futile efforts to change can be fulfilled by all those methods which, when effective, alter a client's view of reality. These include facilitating insight, interpretation, redefinition of a problem, reframing, cognitive restructuring, imagery techniques, covert sensitization and desensitization, modeling, use of metaphor, and storytelling. These methods attempt to alter the client's concepts, expectations, beliefs, views of reality, world view, or guidelinies for behavior. In addition to providing a map or path for change (which is a separate function described below), these methods can also effectively block previously futile behaviors.

For example, in the case of the wife attempting but failing to cheer up her depressed husband, the problem was redefined by the therapist from depression to irresponsibility. This redefinition altered the wife's view of the problem, which in turn dictated different helping behaviors than she previously used. Instead of attempting to cheer up her husband, she could attempt to teach him responsibility. In the case of a woman who could not control her need for revenge on a man who had jilted her (a loss of control which was so severe that it resulted in repeated acts of vandalism against the man), her vengeful behavior was put to an abrupt end when the therapist reframed this behavior as an excellent way to boost the self image of a man with a fragile sense of masculinity. This reframing did not result in a greater degree of "will power"; she had already been exerting her will power to the utmost. It simply resulted in a different view of reality, a view which no longer dictated vengeful acts as a way of meeting her needs.

Reality is altered in a similar way by interventions which establish a relationship between the client and something (or someone) else, a relationship which is incompatible with the client's relationship to the problem. For example, a negative or confictual relationship can be established between the client and some aversive event which outweighs or is more important than the client's conflictual relationship with the problem. Ordeal therapy (Haley, 1984) and punishment methods derived from behavior therapy can accomplish this by making some ordeal or aversive event contingent on the occurence of the problem behavior. This blocks, or contracts and cuts short, the problem maintaining behaviors.

For example, when an alchoholic is taking antabuse (which causes violent illness upon intake of alchohol) or when a smoker has commited himself to an ordeal after each cigarette, the ruminations and conflict about whether or not to smoke or drink are cut short. There is no contest between the relationship with violent illness and the relationship with whether or not to drink. To drink or not is no longer worth the asking. The client finally lets go of, drops, is distracted from, or forgets the painful conflict with the ordeal, and in the process automatically lets go of the symmetrical conflict with the problem. The ordeal interupts the feedback loop described by Bateson in which a person repeatedly attempts to verify that a certain behavior leads to discomfort; it interupts it by verifying this with emphatic punctuation, but on *this* side of death.

Positive relationships also serve the same blocking functions. These relationships can be those formed between client and therapist and with others. A good therapeutic example is that of helping a client to develop a growing commitment to the relationship between himself and his body so that the client's relationship with a problem (such as smoking) becomes less important in comparison; that is, the urge to smoke is not denied but becomes "odd man out." This effectively blocks attempts to "try not to smoke", attempts which are likely to maintain the problem.

Conveying the Message that Change will Occur

The second function fulfilled by various therapeutic methods is that of fostering the belief that change will occur. This function is fulfilled by most of the methods mentioned above which aim to alter a client's view of reality. In addition to the function of blocking problem-maintaining efforts to change the problem, they sometimes provide models and guidance for more effective behavior which the client believes has a high probability of effecting change; in addition to fostering this belief, these methods in themselves may actually effect change.

Another class of methods includes paradoxical interventions and prescriptions of family rules which have been maintaining problems. In addition to serving the function of blocking problem-maintaining efforts at change which was noted above, they convey the implication that the effort to produce the problem with deliberation or in a different interpersonal field can result in a diminution of the problem.

Induction of a convincing trance is a powerful way of conveying the message that therapeutic change will occur. When a client is convinced that he or she has experienced a trance or a hypnotic response, then the client is likely to believe that the hypnotist's methods will reduce the problem about which the client complained. Hence, the value of trance induction procedures, deepening techniques, and methods which ratify for the client the occurence of trance.

One method that is rather constant across all forms of therapy is the creation of a situational and interpersonal context that conveys the message that change will occur. This context is created by the very act of the client walking into the therapist's office (rather than the therapist seeking out the client), by the therapist collecting a fee (rather than paying the client), and by the therapist setting another appointment. Even when the therapist has verbally told the client that he is not sure he can help (which is a "don't change" message conveying the therapist's impotence), the act of collecting a fee and setting another appointment carries the implication that coming to therapy will result in change.

A sense of hope and expectancy of change, generated by the therapist's demeanor and attitude, can have a contagious effect and foster expectancy, hope, and belief in the client that change will occur. Anything a therapist does or any advice a therapist gives can constitute an implicit message that by doing "such and such", change will occur. The "such and such" may consist of injunctions to free-associate, listen to interpretations, engage in empty-chair psychodramas, talk about feelings, draw genograms, or for father and son to spend some extra time together washing the car.

A related method by which this message is conveyed is the practice of ritual, that is to say, some sequence of procedures which the therapist indicates will cause change to occur. A characteristic of ritual is that its effective ingredients are to some degree incomprehensible to the client. Rather than detracting from the efficacy of ritual, this characteristic of incomprehensibility actually enhances the belief that change will occur by engaging in the ritual because it prevents the client from analyzing the dubious causal link between the ritual and the effect of change it is presumed to cause.

Many hypnotic techniques utilize ritual in the way just described. For example, ritual is used in this way every time a hypnotist makes statements of the following form; "As you slowly count to ten, your eyelids will feel heavier and heavier." There is no actual causal connection between counting to ten and eyelids becoming heavier, but the use of causal connectives such as the word "as" in the above quote convey the implication that engaging in a particular behavior has properties, incomprehensible to the client, which will cause certain hypnotic or curative effects. It should be noted that the incomprehensibility of the causal connection facilitates the belief in change only when, paradoxically, the ritual has an overiding appearance of validity.

Moving only a step or two away from ritual, it can be seen in hypnotic suggestions that the causal portions of the suggestions (beginning with words like "If" or "As" or "When") are equivalent to statements made by skilled hypnotists which "pace" or mirror the client's current experience and invoke truisms, all of which the client cannot dispute. Examples include "As you listen to my voice . . . . " or "While you sit there and notice that you have certain feelings . . . . " or "Because you have struggled so long and hard with this conflict . . . ." The rapport that is established by these sensitive, empathic, and indisputable statements lead the client to blur the distinction between these causal statements and the second portion of the suggestion, that is, the leading suggestions for change. Examples of the second portion include " . . . . you may notice your eyelids becoming heavier" or " . . . . you may have already begun to notice a change in your attitude towards this conflict you have been struggling with."

An example of a complete suggestion of this kind, containing both causal and effect portions, is as follows: "As you notice that you have certain feelings while you sit there, you can notice certain changes in them.'' When pacing and leading occur in a way in which it is difficult to differentiate between the two processes there are two results: a message is conveyed that change will occur and actual change usually occurs which ratifies the belief that change will continue to occur.

The sensitive pacing just described is accomplished in all forms of therapy which utilize methods of active listening, reflective listening, ''joining'' with the client, or establishing rapport, such as in structural family therapy, nondirective play therapy, and client-centered counseling. With the exception of structural therapy, these therapies emphasize the pacing rather than leading aspect and may even attempt to avoid the leading aspect. Yet, leading is inescapable; it is implicit in the therapy situation and is also unwittingly accomplished when therapists selectively attend to changes which they believe to constitute growth.

These methods and those described in the previous section certainly do not exhaust the ways in which a belief in change can be fostered and conscious efforts to change can be blocked. The reader can consider other therapies and therapeutic methods and derive from them additions to this list of ways in which these two functions are fulfilled.

Extraneous Agents of Change

A variety of potential change agents may have effects not predicted by the two functions, described above, which establish a hypnotic relationship. Nevertheless, these potential change agents do have a place in the application of this approach. Potential agents include possibly valid or efficacious ingredients in any of the therapeutic methods, both those noted above as serving other functions and those not noted here. Some examples include methods of reframing reality, prayer, modeling, use of metaphor, hypnotic suggestion which may mobilize an internal restructuring in clients, the teaching of etiquette, restructuring relationships, breaking alliances, fostering alliances, triangulation, realigning hierarchies, free association, God, cognitive restructuring, Ritalin, massage, and so on.

It is not a function of this model to either denigrate, advertise, or otherwise comment on which of these various potential agents of change may actually have impact on problems. This judgement is one which each therapist must make on the basis of his or her training, knowledge of human behavior and the sciences, familiarity with outcome research, years of experience, and individual belief system. In view of conflicting research results and an immortal controversy concerning which of these potential change agents are more or less effective if effective at all, it is impossible for me to believe that I can rely soley on any of these potential agents as vehicles for therapeutic change. Belief in the efficacy of these potential agents, or use or invocation of them, is not necessary to facilitate change according to the assumptions of the model articulated here. I believe that change can be accomplished or facilitated soley by the establishment of an interpersonal context, of a specific form, which maximizes the probability of change. Yet, it would be foolish to avoid using those potential change agents in which, by experience or belief or acquaintance with research, one has developed confidence as having some likelihood of facilitating change. Use of these may enhance the change process.

For optimal effect it may sometimes be necessary that clients be distracted from these change agents so that the clients do not engage in efforts which interfere with the efficacy of these agents or to allow the time necessary to elapse for an impact to occur. For example, a hypnotic suggestion for relaxation or glove anesthesia may require time for internal processes to mobilize the required response, in as yet unknown ways. A massage used as one of several methods to reduce a headache may lose efficacy if the client's critical attention is placed upon it as a possible causal agent. The value of a spontaneous discovery by spouses that they are enjoying each other's company on a long-overdue date prescribed by the therapist may be diluted if they focus their attention on this date as being a primary agent of change. A reduction of caffeine intake could lose its critical importance in the change process of a client with panic attacks if the client believes that this was the only crucial factor of importance. In each of these cases, some degree of distraction may be necessary to maximize the impact of potential change agents.

Distraction

Distraction or redirection of attention plays an important function in the coherence of this approach despite being discussed last. As mentioned earlier, when only a minimal degree of distraction exists the interaction is not usually recognized as hypnotic, but it is only this minimal degree that is usually necessary to accomplish most therapeutic goals. First, distraction helps at times to preserve the message that change will occur because this message may be in the form of a very questionable suggestion. Numerous methods are useful for distracting the client from the dubious logic inherent in the therapeutic suggestion that by virtue of the occurence of some presumed cause (e.g., coming to sessions weekly, free-associating, counting from one to ten, etc.), some desired effect will result (e.g., arm levitation, improved family functioning, self actualization, etc.).

Distraction prevents a person from examining each therapeutic suggestion with the same critical and skeptical attitude that he might bring to bear on other issues of everyday life. It helps the client to "suspend disbelief" which permits a certain degree of acceptance of reality distortion, such as for hallucinations or for less unusual changes. Once some amount of change has occured, it is useful to allow, or redirect, the client's attention to be placed on this change, so that it can be verified as occuring, but then is sometimes best to redirect it away once again so that the change can continue unimpeded by the client's critical attention.

Many examples of this form of distraction exist in the practice of hypnosis; since it may be more difficult to illustrate in the more general practice of therapy, an example of the latter is given here. When an individual notices that he hasn't experienced an urge to smoke for a few days or even for a few hours, attention to this matter not only pleases the individual but may also occasion some dissonance, disorientation, or confusion. The person has been a smoker for so long that he now feels disoriented and confused about who he is since he no longer wants to smoke.

This disorientation can lead him to restore his sense of the continuity of self by developing an urge to smoke once again, because the smoking habit helps him to keep track of who he is. It is useful to guard against this eventuality by predicting the disorientation as normal, which implies that there is no need to study and comprehend it, an implication which directs attention elsewhere at the same time that it confirms the reality of change. In this example, it can be seen that distraction also serves to facilitate the perception that behavior is involuntary, that is, that change is occuring on its own without a struggle.

In the same way that distraction from a change agent may help to preserve the efficacy of that agent, distraction can be used to help block a client's conscious efforts to change; this function was noted earlier as being equivalent to the message "Don't try to change." In addition, further distraction can help preserve the efficacy of previous maneuvers to distract or block a client from problem maintaining efforts. This consists of distraction from distraction. For example, in asking a child who hallucinates voices, voices which tell her not to listen to the therapist, to stop trying to prevent the hallucination and instead to go ahead and have one (which is a maneuver intended to distract her from or block previous efforts to avoid hallucinations), it might very well be necessary to distract her by some additional maneuver from the fact that it is the therapist who is asking her to have the hallucination.

Even if this situation was less confusing in the paradoxical sense by, for example, the child having painful headaches instead of hallucinations, the risk exists that maneuvering her into giving up efforts to avoid headaches by attempting to have them might be met with genuine fear of pain. It is also possible that this or other prescriptions to give up struggling could remind her that she must give up struggling, a reminder difficult to forget and which could lead her to struggle with the question of whether to struggle or not, which is an easy path back to her original struggle with the problem. It would be useful to attach some additional purpose to the prescription which blocks struggling with the problem in order to distract her from the injunction not to struggle. For example, she could be given the distracting rationale that to bring on a headache is the first step in controlling it or that it is better to ambush a headache when well rested and prepared than to be ambushed by it when caught unawares.

Finally, methods of distraction can increase the probability that clients will feel compelled to respond to both levels of the bi-level message conveyed by the therapist. They help to prevent a client who is capable of mental acrobatics from formulating conclusions which would allow him to recognize the therapist's bi-level, paradoxical message and to comment on this message at a meta-level. For example, the client might laugh at, express annoyance at, or otherwise comment on the double bind into which the therapist was attempting to place him.

It may appear that there is something deceptive about methods of distraction described here and it is true that distraction can be used with deceptive intent. However, it can be effectively used, in the ways described here, even after these ways have been fully explained to someone. As was pointed out earlier, distraction is employed in this way, successfully, by anyone using self hypnosis. It is not the individual that is tricked or deceived but rather the cognitive equipment which we all share. Distraction is successful, despite knowledge of its use, because it capitalizes on a human limitation, the limitation on the number of perceptions or thoughts one can attend to at a given point in time.

Summary of the Model

The model describes a specific form of therapeutic interaction with clients and proposes that this form of interaction consists of an interpersonal context that is optimal for facilitating change in many instances. The context can be described most clearly by language which specifies a peculiar set of relationships between therapist, client, and problem, and by language which specifies the peculiar sets of messages conveyed by therapist and client.

Using relationship terminology, it is proposed that the client's symmetrical struggle with a problem is altered when the client is maneuvered into a surrender in regard to the struggle, a maneuver which is accomplished by the therapist preventing the client from defining the therapeutic relationship as either symmetrical or complementary. Using communicational terminology, the client's complaint, from a one-down position, conveys helplessness, a message which indicates that he is not producing the problem, at least not purposely. This message is incongruous with the message conveyed by the problem itself, namely, that the client is indeed producing it. This paradoxical message is structurally equivalent to that conveyed by any hypnotic response. Therefore, the therapist can interlock and gain leverage on this response by treating it as a hypnotic one, that is, by conveying a paradoxical message in return.

He does this by conveying and fostering the belief that change will occur. Yet, he sidesteps or avoids insistence on this belief when the client indicates that the problem is too powerful to control. Thus, he avoids a competitive struggle with the client. He does this at the same time that he conveys the message that the client cease all deliberate efforts to try to directly solve the problem. In this way he prevents a relationship being established in which the client obediently tries to will away the problem and fails. Instead, the therapist gives the client something else to do.

This something else may consist of behaviors which block or prevent the kinds of conscious struggle and deliberate efforts which would maintain the problem. These behaviors might consist of efforts to bring on the problem, free-association, behavioral methods, chit-chat between therapist and client, or the practice of exotic and incomprehensible rituals. Whatever this something consists of, it conveys the implication that by virtue of this something's occurence (e.g., a ritual), change will occur. Engaging in this behavior also serves to distract the client from the message that change will occur, allowing time for this message to take hold.

Further methods of distraction can also be applied to ensure that while the client is being enjoined both to change and to not try to change he will neither examine the dubious logic of the causal assumption inherent in the suggestion for change nor respond on a meta-level to the paradoxical injunction. The client can then respond paradoxically by changing but indicating in some way that he is not changing on purpose; rather, that it is happening effortlessly, with the struggle left behind.

To back up a bit, if the therapist believes that other potential change agents can augment the impact on the problem and facilitate change, these too can be applied. In applying these agents, the therapist may wish to distract the client from them. As change occurs, the therapist can allow the client to notice it, or direct his attention to it, in order to verify its validity and increase the belief that change will occur. However, the therapist may find it useful to again redirect or distract attention from this change to prevent the kind of critical examination that could lead to a resumption of the client's efforts at deliberate change.

Final Comments on the Model

The relevance of this model to therapy is illustrated in the next section of the book by numerous case examples. Each case is approached somewhat differently, which may sometimes distract the reader from a more general understanding of the model's application. Some general comments will be made in the remainder of this chapter on strengths and weaknesses of the model, on therapist maneuverability, and on the fact that this model only constitutes a particular way of defining reality.

One useful aspect of the focus on therapeutic stance is that it simultaneously sensitizes the therapist to the value of sophisticated techniques and to the value of establishing a specific sort of therapeutic relationship. An implication of this statement is that techniques, no matter how sophisticated, provocative, or "razzle-dazzle," may fail in the absence of the establishment of a particular kind of relationship, and that this relationship by itself establishes an interpersonal and communicational context for change and resolution of problems.

This is an observation that has been made repeatedly, often by older and experienced therapists, from various therapeutic camps (e.g., Bordin, 1979; Hutt, 1976; Hynam, 1981), who have lamented on the ineffectiveness of "techniques" of psychotherapy but who have asserted that there is an elusive something about therapy that is nevertheless of value. They have, in their comments, hinted at one or another of the specific features of the therapeutic relationship which I have attempted here to synthesize into a coherent system. Yet, while the focus here is on the therapeutic relationship, this focus does not preclude the use of techniques, strategic or otherwise, simple or razzle-dazzle. It even sensitizes one to ways of augmenting the effectivenss of techniques.

The model provides a skeletal structure for therapeutic interaction which the therapist can rely on for guidance as to why his intuition is telling him that things "feel right" or "feel wrong." It can alert the therapist to many of his own and his clients maneuvers which threaten to impede change. For example, if the therapist feels he has not been helpful in a particular session and succumbs to this feeling, he might make the mistake of not collecting a fee or not setting another appointment. In a situation like this the collection of a fee or the setting of another appointment might be the only means left for the therapist to convey to the client the message that change will occur. Failing to convey this message at some level defeats the purposes of both client and therapist. By leaning on this model, the therapist can, in a situation like this, feel confident that he is still doing a good job by simultaneously conveying the message that change will occur (perhaps by nothing more than fee collection and the setting of another appointment) and conveying the message that things look bad; so bad that it might be impossible for him to ever figure out what is wrong or do anything to be helpful though he is willing to try if that is satisfactory to the client. As has been suggested by others (e.g., the MRI group), announcing one's impotence in this way can help more than hurt the process of therapy.

This example in which the therapist takes a predominantly pessimistic view about change does not imply that pessimism is the preferred view dictated by the model. In many cases it is useful to take a predominantly optimistic and hopeful view, in order to instill positive expectancy and to foster the belief that change will occur. For example, in hammering out the details of a complicated behavioral plan involving a system of reinforcement contingencies, there might evolve, in therapist, parents, and children, a growing confidence in the probability of success. This can be useful, as long as at some level the message is still conveyed that change may not be possible. The parents may have stopped receiving that latter message if at the end of the session they ask if the therapist can now assure them of problem resolution within the next two weeks. Leaning on the model, the therapist is able to be alert to this complementary maneuver and make clear that there are no guarantees.

Another example is that of clients attempting to define the therapeutic relationship by requesting weekly or bi-weekly appointments at a particular time of day. This is understandable in terms of the client's need to make logistical arrangements of convenience, and the therapist can accept such requests if they do not threaten his leverage in being the one to define the relationship. Yet, he must be prepared to refuse this request or modify the schedule, especially if he does not yet know enough about the problem to know what he might want to do about it and finds that the type and frequency of treatment is being dictated by the client.

These comments are not meant to exhaust the topic of therapist maneuverability. Fisch et al. (1982) have provided a greater number of more innovative suggestions on therapist maneuverability, which, incidentally, summarize suggestions made by numerous others in the literature. Yet, the preferred stance in most of their suggestions is that of cautious pessimism. This reflects only one level of the bi-level message conveyed by therapists. Optimism is also frequently appropriate.

Also, the book "Paradox and Counterparadox," written by the Milan group (Palazzoli et al., 1975) is replete with similar rationales for procedures aimed at achieving and maintaining therapeutic leverage. Their rationales for procedures may be more useful to therapists in general than the procedures themselves. The procedures they have gradually developed to maintain this therapeutic leverage have taken on a rigidity which, in my own experience, actually limits maneuverability; they might even impede a therapist working without the help of a co-therapist and a consultation team. The purpose of including the few comments here on this topic is to illustrate the wider range of maneuverability that is possible when the parameters of a paradoxical therapeutic stance are explicit to the therapist.

Another interesting feature of this model is that the paradoxical injunction to clients which it prescribes reflects a therapist position which preserves the therapist from disappointment when clients fail to change, yet maximizes the therapist's ability to wait for or to leverage a change. That is, the position is one in which the therapist can recognize at all moments in all cases that it is quite possible that helping the client to change may not be within the therapist's control or grasp, and that whatever feats he performs may not matter in the least. Yet, even with this pessimistic view, he simultaneously takes action which conveys an optimistic message. That is, he acts as if what he is doing will matter and he uses all the knowledge at his disposal on the chance that some piece of it will happen to make a difference.

By taking this paradoxical position he remains less invested in the outcome of therapy than in assuring the quality or process of the therapy. To many therapists, when therapy is conducted in this way, it tends to feel "right" or "special" and worth each moment for its own sake. When conducted in this way, it may increase the chances of positive outcomes even though the emotional investment is less on outcome than on the action of the moment.

As a conceptual framework, the model contains a particular weak point. This Achilles' heel is in the consideration given to potential change agents extraneous to the model but which are usable within its framework. The consideration given to these potential change agents carries the implicit recognition that any of these agents could possibly render effective, be just as effective, or be more effective than those features specified as more central to the model. Yet, this weak point may not be so very damaging.

After all, this model only reflects an attempt to describe an interpersonal context for change which the therapist can establish, and cannot presume to be a description of the only mask of truth about change. This weak point may be a useful source of strength in that it provides an open invitation for a revision of the model, perhaps a more refined and more logical restructuring of concepts. In such a revision, certain ideas might be redefined or relegated to a different status, but essential meanings in the interrelationships of ideas could be preserved.

Another source of strength in this weak point is that it liberates a therapist to use any method he or she wishes without robbing that method of its uniqueness, or denying or diluting the validity of its theoretical underpinnings. In this way, a therapist remains free to use behavioral, analytic, pharmacological, or other approaches, appreciating the differences among theoretical frameworks and recognizing the probability that each can be powerfully applied in given conditions. This freedom is constrained only in the sense that whatever the therapist does will make sense from at least one constant point of view, the view of the therapeutic relationship that has been articulated here. This view can innoculate the therapist from the paralysis of confusion that is sometimes occasioned by shifting from the assumptions of one method or model to another. Instead, it can encourage the kind of rapid shifting from model to model that renders an eclectic approach efficient and sensible, rather than a chaotic use of a grab-bag of techniques.

Concluding Remarks

In view of some of the more sophisticated models of therapeutic change currently undergoing development, the model articulated here might be better viewed as a crude set of practical guidelines and handy observations which have been helpful to some therapists in organizing a vast array of therapeutic phenomena. It has been necessary to articulate something of this kind because I, as well as many others, wish to use in a sensible way and on a practical level the many similarities in technique noticed in the practices of healers of all kinds. These include hypnotists, behaviorists, analysts, Rogerians, gestaltists, Jungians, cabalists, witchdoctors, and wise old grandmothers.

It is what we have noticed in the practices and explanations of practicioners and theoreticians that constitutes the model articulated here. This is especially the case in regard to the concept of the therapeutic doublebind formulated by those associated with the Bateson project. As its parameters have been fleshed out and been made increasingly evident in diverse therapeutic applications, I have noticed that it imposes a view on reality; and thus far (though this may change) it has been a view which I think has increased by own and other therapists' efficiency.

If there is no such thing as paradox except in the mind of the therapist, as some have suggested, then that fact invalidates the very foundations of this model except insofar as a reality in the mind of a therapist can have therapeutic impact. While a model of reality is not reality itself, it has some relative utility in negotiating with reality. I have found this model useful in negotiating the reality of therapeutic change and think it might be useful to others, even if its value is akin to Don Quixote perceiving an ordinary windmill and believing that a malevolent sorceror has transformed himself into the appearance of an ordinary windmill.

Yet, maintaining the distinction between model and reality is difficult when we attempt to describe either reality or our models of it. Communication requires a choice and a utilization of concepts which immediately distort and limit one's view and which lead inevitably to some degree of reification of the concepts one is using. Commission of this error to some extent is inescapable in any act of explication, just as it was inescapable for Don Quixote and the characters with whom he interacted. It is useful to accept this, and therefore equally useful to remind both myself and the reader that no concept or model can constitute the final face of truth. In accepting this, we then free ourselves to use words and concepts to create whatever realities are most interesting and useful to us at each moment. It is interesting in this regard to recall that even the *Lau Tsu,* which attempts to describe *the* way of viewing reality, begins by saying that '' . . . . the way that can be spoken of is not the constant way.''

PART 2

CASE ILLUSTRATIONS

6

AN INTERVENTION FOR SMOKING: TRANSCRIPT OF A CASSETTE TAPE

As the title indicates, this chapter illustrates an intervention which was applied to the problem of smoking. There is a danger that its placement at the beginning of the case illustrations may reinforce a common but mistaken assumption that hypnotic methods are most appropriate for problems of smoking and overeating. In my experience, these problems constitute only a small minority of the problems presented to therapists and for which hypnotic methods are appropriate, as will become evident as the reader proceeds through subsequent chapters. This intervention for smoking is placed at the beginning of the case illustrations because, out of all the illustrations, it may be the most comprehensive single application of the ideas expressed in Chapters Four and Five. Since it follows on the heels of those more theoretical chapters, the running commentaries which appear in transcripts of subsequent chapters have been omitted here. Commentary is less necessary because the close identities between the ideas expressed here and in previous chapters are more readily apparent.

The individual for whom the intervention was applied had been a heavy smoker for over twenty years. Over the years he had attempted several smoking control programs and methods, but he had never experienced more than a few hours of relief from the problem. It is difficult to say why he could not overcome this problem when useful methods and skilled professionals had been available to him. Perhaps he simply had not been ready or sufficiently motivated to give up the struggle with smoking. He was also a psychologist and a hypnotist who was familiar with the therapeutic approach articulated here.

A cassette tape was designed as the primary means of intervention, which appears on Side 1 of the tape accompanying this book. The transcript of this tape constitutes the bulk of the present chapter. Although the tape was intended as a comprehensive application of the therapeutic approach described in the two previous chapters, it was also tailored to the individual's unique interests, philosophical bent, world view, and goals. Therefore, it is not appropriate for just anyone with a smoking problem. For example, some of its content would be experienced as needlessly aversive to certain people. It would also be experienced as excessively philosophical to some.

The basic intervention contained in the tape is a bi-level message: the smoking problem will go away, but do not try to not want to smoke. The ways in which these messages are conveyed are different in this case than in other cases. As discussed more fully in previous chapters, this bi-level message would be enough to effect change if it could be guaranteed that the individual would attend to it at all points in time, but it can be more easily guaranteed that he would be distracted from it at various points. In order to establish a bi-level message which resonates throughout the different contexts of an individual's experience, it is useful to bind a person in additional ways to an orientation which prevents him from efforts to stop trying not to smoke. The ways this is best done varies from person to person. For some, frequent utilization of self hypnosis rituals is an appealing and effective method. For others, ordeals are particularly appropriate.

Ordeals entail some inconvenient activity as the price for engaging in the problem behavior. When the price is high enough, it simply is not worth smoking, or even worth debating the question of whether to smoke or not to smoke. An example of one type of ordeal is to ask the smoker to feel free to smoke but to keep the cigarettes in the attic or out in the car and to smoke only in that place whenever he wants a cigarette. Another type of ordeal involves improvement in some other area. For example, the smoker could be asked to feel free to smoke but to clean a room after each cigarette, or to practice his handwriting in order to improve it, or to get five minutes of paperwork completed, or engage in some other desired but avoided goal. The smoker is double bound into one or the other kind of improvement. If smoking continues, it at least leads to some other positive effect.

A third type of ordeal, which additionally doublebinds the smoker, is possible if some activity can be identified which precedes smoking and leads to it, or some activity which is avoided by smoking. A good example is a situation in which the smoker is weight conscious and vain about appearance, enjoys a cigarette after eating, and often smokes to avoid eating (as well as for other reasons). The smoker can be asked to feel free to smoke as much as she wishes but to have a doughnut or the equivalent of 150 calories within two minutes following each cigarette (and to carry small but highly caloric candies on her person so that the ordeal is portable and applicable at all times). The meaning of the eating, and its enjoyment, is altered when its transactional function has been redefined and reordered. That is, it is likely to be experienced as odious, or as an ordeal. It is possible in a case like this to not only stop smoking but to also lose the taste for previously cherished doughnuts and sweets.

In all of these cases of ordeal, the smoker is being asked to form a relationship with the ordeal which becomes more powerful than the relationship with the conflict of whether to smoke or not. It is more powerful because the ordeal is more immediately painful or inconvenient than is the struggle with smoking. Rather than struggle with the question of whether to smoke or not, the ordeal comes to predominate in the smoker's ruminations and debates with himself.

Even when the relationship with the ordeal is fairly symmetrical (because the smoker continues to smoke for awhile), it is more inconvenient than the previous struggle with the urge to smoke and will bring about surrender sooner. When the relationship with the ordeal is complementary, it is because the ordeal is so noxious that the thought of it severely contracts any debate, or even nips it in the bud. The smoker may continue to want to smoke, but no longer want to do so enough to do it; that is, he wants to avoid the ordeal more than he wants to smoke. He then simply becomes distracted more frequently from wanting to smoke and experiences the change as effortless. The only voluntary effort required is that of religiously engaging in the ordeal.

Although the problem of smoking can sometimes be addressed briefly and concretely with some of the above approaches, the individual for whom the tape was designed did not want what he described as "doughnut therapy." He had struggled for so long with the problem that he felt it to be a part of his identity; he desired a way to stop smoking that would preserve this side of himself in a way that felt personally meaningful to him. He wished to view and use the resolution of the problem as a progressive step in his personal growth. Therefore, the intervention redefined the problem, the urge to smoke, as a way of accessing a preferred view of reality. It suggested the development of a positive relationship between the individual and his body and with a particular way of viewing reality that the individual considered an accurate or honest view. It combined this with several ordeals which were suggested to occur on a cognitive level rather than in physical action, as will be apparent. Readers who are more interested in family and couple therapy sessions rather than individual work may wish to skip to chapters containing those kinds of case illustrations.

The complete transcript of the tape appears below for those who do not possess the accompanying tape. As will be evident, suggestions for formal trance induction were not provided. Although the tape is sprinkled with some forms of hypnotic language usage and hypnotic suggestions, it generally contains blunt, straightforward language and an abundance of direct suggestions. It utilizes methods taken from direct hypnotic approaches (e.g., Spiegal, 1970) and nonhypnotic therapies, as well as indirect Ericksonian forms.

Transcript of the Tape

As you listen to this tape, you can discover knowledge which you already possess that can enable you to deal with this problem of smoking a bit differently than before. All you need to do is to listen and to allow yourself to effortlessly think thoughts and feel feelings, whatever they are. And in doing this, you can discover things in yourself that lead you to want other things more than you want to smoke. And if your attention wanders from what's being said, there may be good reason for it, and you don't need to worry about it. Your attention can wander back again, and if you've missed anything of importance, you can just listen to the tape again.

Since you've already tried to stop smoking, I don't think you want me to tell you to simply try harder. I won't ask you to do that. Wanting to smoke or not wanting to is involuntary, and you can't make it happen by a voluntary choice. In fact, I'd like to ask you to do the opposite, to preserve your urge to smoke, to be aware of wanting to smoke. Rather than avoid cigarettes, go ahead and touch them, smell them, spy out cigarette butts on the ground, and go ahead and wish for a cigarette as much as you like.

And when you notice that you want to smoke, you can begin to notice how much you want to, even if it takes only a split second to notice. Just checking to see if wanting to smoke is minimal, or if it's urgent, and if other more important wants might also exist alongside it. And if you find, even in that split second, that you definitely want to enough to light up, then feel free to go ahead and light up. You don't have to fight against it. Rather than even debate the question of whether you should or shouldn't have a cigarette, please feel free to go right ahead.

But when you do light up and smoke, do it thoroughly. Place as much of your attention on it as you can. The ideal situation would be to do nothing else while smoking. No television, no writing, no talking, no drinking, no nothing. So that you can place your undivided attention on smoking. That way you can try to extract all the enjoyment that's there. Make it really worth it, because it's at the expense of certain things.

You might begin to realize these expenses when you realize that your enjoyment of the cigarette is not as great as you thought even though you try to enjoy it all you can. You may also realize that what you're doing is attempting to enjoy smoking at the expense of your body. You know certain things about your body that you may not have fully appreciated yet. For one thing, do you realize that your body is helpless and depends on you, like a loved pet, or a plant, or a baby, or a child? How it's cared for is your decision and depends on what you want for it. It depends on your good judgement. Your body is helpless and has no choice but to accept what you put into it. You can put poison into it. Or you can nourish it. That's entirely up to you. When you treat it like a valued pet or a child that you love, then you'll exercise it and feed it properly, and rest it, with the result that it can grow strong and can serve as a good ally to you. Would you put poison into the food of a child, or pet, or an ally?

In thinking about this, can you see that there's a part of yourself that truly wants to care responsibly for your body? Simply because your body is helpless and depends on what you do for it. This caretaker in you views the world honestly and with humility, recognizing that pets and children and bodies are all quite fragile and in need of care in a harsh and unpredictable world that can hurt them. Look at your hands, a part of your body, to realize how strong and wonderful, yet how fragile and in need of care your body is. You already know that if you mistreat it enough, it'll grow sick and experience pain and die and then you'll have it no longer.

And do you see how this can bring you to realize that you need your body? Not only does your body need you and depend on you for its exercise, rest, and care, but you also need your body to live. Do you really understand that you depend on it? You depend on it to experience life. It is only through your body that you experience life, that you see things, feel things, think things, get things done. You ride on it through life as on a pet horse or an automobile. It needs you for its care, and you need it to experience life.

✓ Maybe you don't fully realize yet that this interdependent relationship in which you depend on your body and it depends on you is the single most important relationship in your life. As you develop this relationship with your body, what you want for it can come to outweigh your wanting to smoke. You can begin to feel greater appreciation of this relationship with your body and discover the development in yourself of a growing commitment to this relationship the more you find yourself thinking about it whenever you feed your body, dress it, exercise it, take it for a walk, or rest it. And how long do you think it will take to begin to notice this relationship when your body allows you to enjoy a taste, or to see something interesting, or to do a job, or to think? How long before you recognize this relationship in anything you do? When you really realize that this is the single most important relationship in your life, it can change everything for you.

✓ How can you truly know how to care for others, which requires a respect for their need for care, unless you can recognize and respect your own body's need for care? You can act like you care for others, but can you really respect and understand their need for care without respecting your own need for care?

✓ This recognition and respect for your body's need for care is a powerful way of viewing things because it involves the perception that your body is fragile, that it's at the mercy of unpredictable catastrophes, that it's mortal, a hollow reed in the wind, and that it will die. This point of view is one which looks death squarely in the face as a reality, not as a fiction, and recognizes that death is working on us even now, and can even strike in the next few moments, and is always with us. This is a viewpoint which can accept the dark side of life and recognize the misery in the world, which can acknowledge the drudgery, the boredom, the pain, the feelings of emptiness and loneliness, and really see how little control and understanding of things we really have. This is an acceptance of the inevitable pain in life.

This more honest view of things is a frightening one. When some feeling of drudgery or some other pain occurs that reminds us of this dark side of things which we do not wish to see so vividly, we find many

ways to distract ourselves from it. And when we fly from it, we manufacture unnecessary pain, in millions of ways which are at the expense
of others and at the expense of ourselves as well. But when we can
tolerate viewing this dark side, accepting even the reality of death, for
only the few moments it takes to feel exactly how horrible things really
are, we can find in that acceptance an interesting strength.

The recognition of the reality of death is a recognition that each of
your actions could be your last action. This can lead you to give each
moment its due respect and can guide you to be at your best, to take the
very best action available to you. It can guide you to take responsible
action and to take responsibility for each of your acts. It can nurture the
growth of a commitment and a relationship between you and your body
and can also guide you to a respectful relationship towards all other things
as well. Do you know that paradise is regained when you step into
harmony with things and with yourself in this way? And that paradise
is lost again as soon as you step out of harmony by running from this
harsh reality, by denying how ignorant and weak you are. By pridefully
acting as if you know more than you do and are more powerful than you
really are.

DR ✓Few of us enjoy the power that exists in this harsh view of life and
death, because we don't look for the few moments longer it takes to
appreciate this power. As soon as we are really reminded that such a
reality exists, we run from it like a scared child. As soon as we are
reminded of it by any hint of death, by any misery, by any feeling of
being one-down or being deprived, or wanting something like a drink or
a smoke and fearing we won't get it, we don't even hesitate to see what
would happen if we accepted these things. Like children, we fly from
these, turning away and taking a self deceptive and distorted view of
things, like a puffed up child who momentarily believes he is all powerful
and can slay anything and not be slain, wanting so desperately to feel
powerful and one-up on the world. Wanting to feel knowledgable and
not so ingnorant about this incomprehensible world.

To feel one-up like this, we do many things at the expense of others.
We show them how smart we are compared to them, we insult them, we
talk behind their backs, and we even try to teach them when they don't
wish to be taught. And we do things at the expense of our bodies. We
exercise too much or too little, sleep too long or not enough, eat too
much, drink too much, and smoke too much. When we do any of these
things, we act as if we were immortal. We flatter and lie to ourselves
in order to feel self important. By drinking or smoking we are daring

death to be real. And this challenge pleases us. It helps us to deny and
forget the humbling facts of life. For example, the fact that we need this
body to experience life. The scared and foolish child in us tries to deny
this fact by smoking and drinking even more. He tries to poison this body
to verify whether it will really happen, to try to confirm that it won't.
He sucks down a drink or drags on a cigarette as if his body cannot be
harmed by it, as if his body is not needed to experience life. And as he
does so, he struts about and boasts and laughs too loud, enjoying the
image of being important and invincible, enjoying this image at the
expense of his body and at the expense of a more honest view of things.
How long do you think he can go on like this before he can deny reality
no longer? Before the scales fall from his eyes?

The very existence of this more honest view that lies within you is
enough to threaten that child's one-up stance and to create a nagging
doubt that will lead him to challenge and defy reality again and again,
acting as if your relationship with your body were unimportant. This
scared and foolish child in you won't even want to seriously consider the
request that when you smoke you do it thoroughly with undivided attention because in smoking in this way the expenses are far too apparent
and too frightening.

Go ahead and try it. Don't distract yourself, at least just one time. On
lighting up, try to enjoy that one-up stance thoroughly, and focus on
what you are doing by smoking. Say to yourself with the cigarette in
your hand, "I am, with this next drag, trying to poison my body, to see
if I can be immortal and to see if I can deny the notion that my body
depends on me and I depend on it."

Instead of doing this, the scared and foolish child in you will insist on
smoking while typing, smoking while chatting, or smoking while doing
something that distracts from these expenses. This shows just how desperate is the need to distort reality. Think of someone you know who is
the very image of this self deceptive kind of act, puffed up and laughing
too loud and boasting and smoking and drinking and behaving in ways
that makes him feel one-up at the expense of others. Do you realize that
whenever you light up while chatting or typing or doing something else,
you more than ever flatter these people and confirm their view of things?
Do you realize that this person is you whenever you light up while
engaging your attention on another activity? And your one-up act of
lighting up is an agreement with this self deceptive view of things. It's
a confirmation of it. Especially when you give the hollow sound of being
wise and insightful about the world and display the false picture of good
health.

This self deceptive view of things, despite the enjoyment in it of challenging reality, may come to be far more unacceptable and frightening to you than an honest and painful look at things. Which is worse? You think you have a choice, to choose to smoke or not. Look at all you choose when you choose to smoke. Allow yourself again to see the image of that arrogant person. Can you see yourself in that image?

Because from now on, whenever you smoke while chatting, or doing other things, you can no longer entirely escape this image. You can't escape it forever, can you? Go ahead and try to forget that the act of smoking is a self deceptive act of arrogance that is enjoyed at the expense of your body and at the expense of an honest look at life. It will be harder and harder to forget this the more you find yourself committed to a relationship with your body and the more you discover that you can tolerate the recognition of how horrible things can be for the few moments it takes to derive the strength in that recogintion.

The opportunities for the development of this strength are everywhere in daily life. We don't need to wait for a confrontation with death. We need only recognize that it might grab us and those we love at any time. We need only recognize our dissatisfaction with an imperfect world. Or notice a pain or discomfort. Or a rough road. An unfulfilled wish. A feeling of emptiness. A sense of boredom. The raining on a picnic. A wanting to smoke and a fear of being deprived. An insult to our self esteem. Almost anything. These are inevitable pains. Rather than fly from these aspects of the darker side of life, rather than manufacture unnecessary pain, do you realize that you can embrace the inevitable pain in life and appreciate what it can do for you? Can you accept this pain for just long enough for it to show you how wonderful and enjoyable living can be? It can show you the world in a different light and enable you to take humble and responsible action, to do things with respect and care and at no one's expense and to be effortlessly doing the best of which you are capable. You won't come to enjoy pain, but you can come to appreciate it, embrace it, and utilize it as a short pathway to discovering greater value in living.

When you view life and death in this way, you are taking an honest look at things and accepting your own mortality. You're no longer viewing things in a self deceptive intellectualized way in which you continue to smoke and drink while eloquently philosophizing about the face of death, but instead you're viewing things in a real, everday, mundane way. Because the face of death is your own face, your own body. You have only to look at your hands to remind yourself of your body's mortality, and it's inevitable death. How long will it take before noticing your hands, or noticing a one-down feeling, or noticing you want to smoke can be used as a reminder to recognize the pain in life and in that recognition to view things honestly and respectfully.

There are so many reminders in the world, so very many signals that can trigger various chains of ideas you have been thinking about here. Rely on them to occur all around you and within you. Any exercise you do, any pain, any enjoyments your body permits you, the very listening to these words which your body allows you to do. You don't have to look for these reminders to discover that they are working on you to mobilize resources within you that you didn't know were so strong when you notice yourself changing effortlessly. You may wonder when these changes will happen, or how long it will take. Do you know that it's even already happening now? And you don't even need to try to make it happen.

But a confusing thing may also happen. You may change too quickly at times, or too powerfully, and it may surprise you when it happens. It may surprise you to discover that a period of time has passed in which you forgot to have any strong urges to smoke, and this may disconcert you because for so long you've thought of yourself as a smoker and now you wonder who you are. A smoker? Or an ex-smoker? You can, if you wish, feel free to have a cigarette or to struggle with an urge to smoke, if you wish to comfort yourself by defining who you are in this way. But do you realize you don't really need to keep track of who you are?

You can smoke and drink and put people down and keep track of who you think you are in any of these ways. But when you really understand that you don't need to try to do this any longer, you can let go of these efforts and find that you can rely on your capacity for forgetting. This capacity comes from the limit on how many things you can attend to at a given point in time. It can be counted on to distract you from these efforts, if you only let it. Since you can keep only several things in mind at once, things can be easily forgotten. As your attention is distracted to the sound of a car, or drawn to a bird chirping, or to a character's dialogue on T.V., a view out a window, a thought about lunch, or anything else, you may find a remarkable strength in trusting in your ability to become interested in many different things, one after another, and forget to re-member who you are, or forget to remember an urge to smoke. Even as you listen to me you find it difficult at times to remember what I have just said or to keep yourself from becoming distracted by your own thoughts, with your mind wandering here and there.

This happens to us all. We forget all kinds of things but hardly ever do we realize we can use this capacity for our benefit. It is with us all the time, and we need only to allow it to happen. We need only stop trying to remember so hard. We only need to let go, and allow our attention to become interested and drawn to one thing after another, until our attention comes back around and notices, with a pleasant surprise, that it has forgotten the need to smoke, and then to allow it the little time needed to wander off again. This capacity to forget things is one that we all have in great abundance, but one which we complain about instead of letting it work for us.

And as soon as you begin to rely on this capacity you'll notice that you've forgotten, at one time or another, to have an urge to smoke. And you don't have to forget on purpose. Most things that we're good at we don't need to do on purpose. It's impossible for us to act with purpose and with conscious deliberation in more than a very few of the many daily acts of eating breakfast, stepping up a curb, or putting the words of a sentence we are rapidly speaking into a very particular sequence as if the choice of each word in relation to every other was a conscious choice. If it depended on conscious choice, we would never figure out the correct sequence of the first two words and the sentence would never get spoken. We delude ourselves when we remind ourselves, or try to believe, that what we are doing depends on conscious deliberation and trying.

Almost everything we might do can be done better without deliberate and conscious attempts to will it to occur. When one accepts the humbling fact that things get done without one's willing it, one can notice that one's behavior is often effortless behavior; that is, one is certainly producing that behavior but not producing it on purpose or effortfully. The less you try to make things happen with conscious effort, the more things seem to get done effortlessly as in a trance.

Trusting in your capacity to forget or to become interested in other things may be the easiest path to change. But there are other paths that you are noticing as well. For example, when you do remember that you want to smoke and you check to see how much you want to smoke, you can notice with curiosity that this wanting might not be as urgent as you thought and that it represents an opportunity for you to recognize how horrible or unfair life can be. Or you can notice that the wanting is not very important compared to other things that you now want much more, such as wanting to take proper care of a body that is precious to you, or that you want much more to enjoy an honest view of life. The chain of thoughts about the expenses of smoking and self deception and arrogance which are evoked by wanting to smoke may soon become painful enough for you to not want to even get started playing those mental games with yourself. I wonder when you'll be ready to simply let go of those games and debates and chains of rumination before they even get going and allow yourself to trust that you can easily become interested in other things.

Our distractible attention has another interesting effect, also disconcerting. That although you may enjoy at this moment a more honest and humble view of things, I can almost guarantee that at some later point, maybe in a couple of seconds, or tomorrow, or next week, you will find that you no longer see things this way. You will have forgotten or become distracted from certain aspects of these ideas that hold them into place so powerfully for you. Or an aspect of it that seems so crucial now, seems less so then. This may seduce you into feeling disappointed and disoriented because you wish to cling to the belief that your view of things and who you are has continuity, and you may then make the mistake of trying to struggle to recapture the preferred view.

You don't really have to try because trying to recapture it prevents all of its aspects from falling into their proper places. This shifting perspective is inevitable because we can only attend to several things at once and at each moment something new occupies our attention and something else leaves it; and in each successive moment we are, in a sense, reborn, reshaped, we are different, and this happens millions of times from one week to the next, from hour to hour, from minute to minute. In an instant, we can correct, distort, or otherwise transform what we are or who we think we are. We can seem to switch right over from one track to a completely different one. You've done it many times. Do you realize that you can just let it happen? You can't stop it from happening, can you? Can an individual wave in a sea of waves be made to retain the same particles of water for more than an instant in time? Do you need to fight it and try to make time and the world stand still?

In noticing that your view of things has shifted and experiencing some sense of wonder at its happening, you can allow it to work for you rather than against you and more rapidly bring back to yourself a more preferred view of things. And this can happen if you don't try to deliberately recapture it and if you learn to be more patient with yourself, as you would with a stubborn, learning child who keeps saying he knows everything you are teaching him.

Sometimes people call this switching back and forth between points of view or tracks of thinking by the name of will power when they are able to stay on the same track for awhile. But the so-called will power involved here is not an act of trying or a struggle. It is an effortless doing of things that comes about through letting go of conscious trying. You don't have to try to will it back. You can simply trust in your own resources to automatically bring it back and to bring about the desired change. Noticing any of the many hints you have been thinking about will do it for you, for example, noticing something unsatisfying about life. You'll find yourself changing and behaving more effortlessly and in desired directions the sooner you stop trying to be a back seat driver telling the driver exactly how far to the right to turn the wheel and exactly how hard to hit the brake. Simply tell the driver where you want him to take you. Isn't this the will power that seems so elusive? It can happen easily if you let it, without a painful struggle, like when you've shifted from second to third gear and find that you can let up on the accelerator and just cruise instead of driving everywhere in second gear.

You sit here now, perhaps convinced of all this, thinking it will be easy. But you may find that you forget it all, especially in the throes of some emotion, or in dealing with a crisis, or while working on some project. You find yourself placing priority on the completion of that activity, and then wonder how you can possibly do it without smoking. Usually you respond to this by forgetting your good resolve and lighting up. I don't want you to think that you have to try to struggle to recapture your resolve in these moments. Instead, I want you now to just take a look at what is happening in these moments.

Your attention has been placed on an outcome, like getting the dishes done so you can watch T.V., or getting that page typed. You have stopped attending to the small pieces of action that go into the doing of the activity or the doing of the chore because there is something about it that you believe to be odious or a drudgery. By keeping your attention on the outcome, for example, what you'll do when you finish the dishes, and distracting yourself from what you do, for example, washing a dish, you act as if what you're doing is an intermission from life, and that mean- ingful life is located somewhere outside of it, and that life will pick up again when you finish the dishes. By defining it in this way, you are the one who makes it a drudgery, you are the one who makes it odious, you are the one who wastes that chunk of your life and destroys it. How many chunks of your life have you been destroying in this way?

You've done this because you've simply forgotten that what you think of as the odious parts of your life are also the living of your life, each moment of those activities. Since you might be struck dead before you finish that chore or activity, you may as well realize that these moments are precious ones too, deserving of their due respect. And who is to say that the act of washing a dish is any less valuable than delivering an exciting speech or hearing a pretty song or having an illuminating insight? Who can presume to make such a judgement? Who can know such a thing? Once you place your attention on the doing of it, you begin to notice what you are doing and no longer are wishing to be away and doing something else. You end up placing attention on aspects thought to be odious but which you now find are not so very odious at all and instead notice interesting things about what you're doing that you didn't notice before. In doing so, you interact with the activity in a different way than before and can thereby find yourself enjoying the interaction and living your life to the fullest.

In order to interact with things in this way, you don't have to try to remember all these things. That would make it more difficult. Instead, you need only remind yourself to slow down, to engage in each action at a rate of speed that is perceptibly slower than usual. This is within your voluntary control and is all you have to do. You will then naturally be placing your attention on what you're doing and will notice yourself viewing your actions differently. You will naturally notice that each moment is the living of your life, and you'll end up paying less attention to what you had wished to do instead. It depends only on slowing down. So instead of saying to yourself, "I can't write without smoking," approach the task of writing differently. Deliberately slow down your physical motions and take pleasure in what you discover about yourself and about writing and about reality.

This may help you to discover a way to utilize that honest and more humble view that you are acquiring, but in everyday activities. It is one thing to view life and death more honestly and with greater humility while sitting in meditation and removed from everyday activity like you are now; it is quite another thing to continue to view things in this way when in the midst of the battles of everyday life, when swept away by the heat of the moment, when trying to fulfill duties and achieve goals. It is too easy to overlook, at these times, the opportunity that exists in the small details of any action, in the means to some end. It is there that one finds the pain and emptiness that brings with it a view of things that is more honest. And one notices that the pain is not so very painful, and that the living of those moments can be quite a bit more interesting than you thought. And you can find that it is not difficult to do this by simply slowing down your action.

Now I don't want you to forget the importance of feeling free to smoke and to feel free to have urges. I think you now know how important they are and that it's better to embrace those urges as useful rather than to fight them. You don't have to even begin to question or debate with yourself about whether to smoke. Simply check to see how much you want to smoke, and if it's enough to do so, you'll know instantly, and you can go right ahead and do it rather than debate about it. But when you decide to do it, enjoy it as thoroughly as you can, attend to it fully if you dare to, and get all there is out of it because that enjoyment has prices which makes the angels weep and which you may try to forget but now will never again be able to deny quite as well as you did before]

Please don't think that you should try to remember all of the many different things you heard and thought about here, nor the interconnections between them. This is not a view of things that you need to try to sustain. It's a view that only needs to be noticed whenever you're ready to notice it. You won't lose it, because each part of it can be accessed by many things. By a problem. By pain. By an urge. The only thing to remember is to feel free to have these pains or these urges and that you don't have to bother to attempt to resist them. If you let them come, then you'll discover ways to let them go]

You can play this tape as much or as little as you like. The more you avoid it, the more painful it probably is to you. The more you play it, the more you can allow yourself to be distracted from one part or another and develop your own reactions, and then come back at another playing of the tape to those aspects from which you were distracted. And all of it can come together in its own time, as your inner resources find the best way to respond and as you learn to depend on them to act for you in all of the various important and trivial moments of the living of your life. It can happen without a painful struggle if you let it. And you can simply notice with pleasure that it's happening, and be patient with yourself when it's not. If you would like, take a few moments before turning off the tape to contemplate any thoughts you feel you need to continue to contemplate.

Concluding Remarks

Although this intervention was tailored to a particular individual, therapists may find it appropriate for other selected individuals. It is more likely, though, that the therapist will need to edit and revise, omitting some parts, expanding other parts, and supplementing the intervention with fresh ideas, in order to adapt it to the purposes at hand.

The primary purpose of this chapter has been to illustrate an intervention which applies as comprehensively as possible the model articulated in Chapters Four and Five. As a consequence, the case description of the individual's problem was brief as were any commentaries and theoretical discussions. In various subsequent chapters, these priorities shift, with emphasis sometimes on case descriptions, sometimes on theoretical discussions, and sometimes on the nonhypnotic therapeutic contexts that surround particular interventions.

7

THERAPEUTIC SUGGESTIONS FOR FORGETTING AN OBSESSION WITH AN EX-LOVER

The application of hypnotic methods in a typical therapy situation is illustrated in the present chapter. The problems consisted of a woman's obsession with an ex-lover and her irresistible compulsion to take vengeance on him. Although the entire course of her therapy is described, the focus is on one particular session. A transcript of that session is provided, with a running commentary explaining the hypnotic methods employed.

The therapeutic purpose of the session was to provide suggestions for a partial amnesia of an obsession. Variations on these suggestions for forgetting have been useful in other cases as well, where it has also been unnecessary to utilize formal trance induction procedures. Since this is an unusual approach to addressing obsessional problems the suggestions for forgetting could be of interest to others. Another interesting feature of this case illustration is that the problem consisted of the wish or compulsion to contact an ex-lover. Difficulty in extricating oneself from self defeating romantic involvements is a very common problem but it is seldom that it receives attention in the psychotherapy literature.

The suggestions for forgetting were not the only effective ingredients in the treatment. They were employed in a context of several other therapeutic interventions which together comprise a package of interventions that have been used to help a number of clients to disentangle themselves from romantic involvements. Although these other interventions fulfill hypnotic functions, they are usually associated with nonhypnotic therapy models. In order to clearly delineate the full clinical context in which hypnotic methods were employed, the transcript is embedded in a case presentation which describes the eight session course of therapy. Theoretical rationales and a comparison to another popular approach to the same problem are provided in the discussion section which follows the case presentation.

The suggestions for forgetting which are detailed in the transcript do not represent much that is new in the hypnosis literature. They include a number of well known Ericksonian techniques which are not always utilized here with the degree of indirection that Ericksonian hypnotists often strive to employ. Yet, the purpose here is not to teach Ericksonian hypnosis as much as it is to illustrate hypnotic methods in a context in which the client does not expect hypnosis and where there is a typical therapeutic utilization of numerous methods which are not ordinarily associated with hypnosis. Readers who are thoroughly familiar with Erickson's methods may therefore find the surrounding therapeutic context to be of more interest than the transcript itself, while nonhypnotic therapists may find the details of the transcript of greater interest.

Case Presentation

Mrs. B., a 26 year old woman, had separated from her husband a year and a half prior to presenting herself for therapy. The separation was due to her need to escape from her husband's domination of her and his insensitivity to her needs. Upon separation, she and her two year old daughter returned to the home of Mrs. B.'s parents where Mrs. B. secured a job in a social work capacity in a state agency. Her husband followed her and the couple began to work towards a reconciliation, still living apart. However, Mrs. B. felt that although her husband was less dominating, he remained insensitive to her needs and did not make her feel "special."

While uncertain about whether to resume living together, Mrs. B. became romantically involved with a man who worked in the same building in which she was employed. Unbeknownst to her husband, she spent a great deal of time in the evenings either with her lover or looking for him. Mrs. B.'s lover was sensitive, empathic, sexually attractive, and was everything she had ever wanted in a man, except in one respect. He frequently battered her and treated her "like a whore," phoning her only when he wanted sex and sometimes kicking her out of his apartment immediately following sexual intercourse. She had tried repeatedly to stay away from him, but, each time she tried, she eventually broke down, called him, and resumed the relationship.

Mrs. B. gradually developed an intense dislike for herself, for allowing herself to be treated in this degrading fashion and for being unable to control herself enough to stay away from this lover. Although she was able to reduce her sexual contacts with him, she developed an intense desire for revenge against him and acted on this desire by making hostile phone calls, smashing his car windows, and having frequent temper tantrums in her parents' home. She could calm herself only by consuming alcohol or tranquilizers. As a result of her distraught condition, her family life with her parents and daughter was in turmoil. She was also very distracted on the job, often breaking into uncontrollable fits of sobbing, and was in danger of losing her position. She felt completely out of control, she worried that she was developing alcohol and drug problems, she feared that she might be arrested for acts of vandalism in any future episodes of loss of control, and both she and her parents believed she was "losing her mind." It was at this point that Mrs. B. called for an appointment.

The history revealed that Mrs. B.'s father, a successful contractor in an upper middle class neighborhood, had ruled the household with an iron hand, playing a very dominating role to his wife's very submissive role. Like her mother, Mrs. B. had learned to play a submissive role and had rarely dared to express any signs of anger or opposition, either to parents or to others. She strived always to please others and this striving seemed to be motivated by a desire to be loved, by fear of abandonment, and a desire to be approved as an adequate and worthwhile person. However, despite her efforts, she could not gain a sense of being approved by her father, nor by her husband, who had also been very critical and domineering, nor by her lover. Her hopes of being approved and loved by types of men who were unlikely to provide complete approval seemed to have driven her to attach herself to such men and attempt to please them.

In the first session, she asked primarily for help in controlling her urge to contact the lover. She feared that she was so much out of control that she would either call him to ask him to have sexual intercourse with her or would commit another act of violence against him or his property which could result in criminal proceedings. In addition, she worried that if she continued to deteriorate, she would never be able to live on her own again. She was asked if she could bring her parents or her husband to the next session but she politely refused this request, saying that she wished to work on the issues of independence and self control outside of the presence of her husband and her parents.

The primary intervention used in the first session was that of reframing her acts of violence against the lover. After she had described something of her lover's character, it was suggested to her in lengthy detail that this man was a person who seemed to feel very inadequate about himself and that he was able to boost his ego and to feel powerful only by degrading Mrs. B. She was told that when she committed acts of violence against him, for example, by making angry phone calls or smashing his car windows, she was mistaken in her belief that she was "getting even with him." Instead, she was "boosting his ego" and "flattering his masculinity and his power over women." Mrs. B. appeared to be stunned by the realization that her efforts to "get even" were producing the opposite effect of boosting her lover's ego.

At the second session two weeks later, Mrs. B. had not contacted her lover and both she and her parents had been relieved to feel a greater sense of control over their lives. Mrs. B. reported that every time she experienced the urge to "get even," she realized that to act on that urge would only serve to boost the ego of her lover. Her consumption of alcohol and medication had also considerably decreased.

However, Mrs. B.'s longing to contact her lover was as pressing as ever. Her hostility and her yearning for him were about equally expressed. In this second session, she was told to go home and to write down, on a single sheet of paper, fragments of all the poignant experiences she could remember of times she had shared with her lover; then she was to spend an hour each evening looking at this sheet of paper, and to listen during this hour to songs which reminded her of her lover. She was told that if she could yearn for him intensely enough during this hour, as well as hate him thoroughly enough, that these feelings might eventually undergo fatigue and be replaced by other feelings. In addition, she was told that if she performed this ritual faithfully, her feelings and ruminations about him would occur less often during the day and would gradually be "contained" within the period of the ritual.

Assertiveness was also discussed in this session because the therapist believed that Mrs. B.'s efforts to please others were maintaining her problems. He suggested to Mrs. B. that if she could learn to be a little more assertive and a little less submissive, she would no longer be putting herself in a position to feel degraded; she could thereby eliminate a source of her explosive anger. He coached her on appropriate assertive behaviors she could try and also employed imagery techniques and cognitive restructuring procedures to help reduce her fear of causing displeasure in others. She was asked to take every opportunity to experiment with being mildly displeasing in safe situations where she would have little to lose, such as with her father.

She was also asked to experiment with "distancing" from others in interactions so that she would not always be at the mercy of her chronic habit of pleasing and "pursuing" others. These tactics will be discussed more fully in the discussion section. Finally, she was strenuously encouraged to throw herself into making a success of a particular project at work which she was in the process of implementing but in which she had not yet emotionally invested herself due to her obsession with her lover.

Mrs. B. dutifully and compliantly followed all suggested tasks in every detail. As a result, she was quite exhausted when she arrived for the third session two weeks later. She had experimented with behaving towards others in displeasing ways and was proud to discover that she could behave assertively. Conflict between she and her parents had increased and she felt proud about this too because it made her feel that she might find the strength to move out on her own if things did not work out with her husband. Mrs. B. had still not contacted her lover and her thoughts about contacting him were occurring less often. The ritual she was performing each night was becoming aversive to her because it was emotionally exhausting to perform.

It was repeated to her at this point that she had previously been violent only because she had not known how to be assertive, and that now that she was becoming increasingly assertive there was no longer a need to be violent. Many other suggestions from the previous session were also repeated, and in general Mrs. B. was told to continue each of the therapeutic tasks. The only additional intervention used in this third session was that Mrs. B. was asked to begin to notice the changes occurring in her life and to begin to wonder where the changes would finally lead.

In the fourth session, two weeks later, Mrs. B. pleaded to be released from her ritual because she was experiencing extreme boredom while performing it. Her yearnings for her lover and her feelings of hostility for him had not entirely disappeared, but they rarely interfered anymore with her daily activities. However, she found that her attention had become dominated by the recurrent thought that she might develop an uncontrollable urge to call her lover. She combated this thought with the resolution to control that urge if it should become too strong. These obsessive thoughts did not seem to be associated any longer with affective features of yearning or of anger.

These thoughts seemed to have the characteristics of a classic obsession. She experienced the thoughts as intrusive, but she did not seem to be in imminent danger of giving in to an urge to contact her lover. Yet her fear of giving in to the urge caused her to obsess more each day about whether she could control the urge if it should grow too strong. The time she spent obsessing was exhausting her, although her daily life had become filled with activities which were now unrelated, either directly or indirectly, to her former relationship with her lover.

In this session, the therapist provided suggestions that would help to distract Mrs. B. from, or help her to forget, her obsession. Mrs. B. knew that the therapist employed hypnotic methods and he had told her in an earlier session that people sometimes go into light trances during therapy. However, the therapist did not say anything in this session about hypnosis. The transcript follows below. It is interspersed with a running commentary which highlights and explains some of the therapist's actions.

Transcript

Therapist: This problem you have, this urge you have, it's in conflict with your efforts to control it. It's like a battle. Control versus urge. The urge isn't strong enough to win over your control of it. But your control isn't strong enough to get rid of the urge. So there you are, always thinking about thoughts of the urge versus thoughts of controlling the urge, thinking and thinking, and exhausting yourself. What a dilemma.

These statements constitute reflective listening. They maintain rapport and serve the hypnotic function of mirroring or pacing the client's current experience.

Mrs. B: You said it.
Therapist: But there is a way out.

This last statement begins to fixate the client's attention by setting up an expectation that something unexpected or unusual is about to occur.

This expectation is analagous to the client's expectation of going into trance when direct methods of hypnosis are employed.

Mrs. B: (*shifts her body positon slightly and becomes more attentive*) There is?
Therapist: It is possible to learn to use our abilities of forgetting, to forget this conflict.
Mrs. B: To forget it?
Therapist: That's right. But it's a trick to do it. You can't just say to yourself, "Oh, I think I'll just forget this problem." No, we do forget to remember many things. But we can't do it on purpose with conscious effort. Consciously we don't have that kind of ability or knowledge. Consciously we don't know very much at all and can't do very much either. For example, you don't know, consciously, whether you're left thumbed or right thumbed (*pause*). Go ahead and clasp your hands behind your head and then look to see which thumb is on top.
Mrs. B: (*Clasps hands behind head and then brings clasped hands in front of her*) My left thumb is on top. Does it mean I'm left thumbed? What does that mean?
Therapist: It means that you have always clasped your hands in this way with the left thumb on top, and that you didn't know this consciously. There are so many things that you have learned and that you know, that are not conscious to you, but you do know them. You see, unconsciously, you knew you were left thumbed. But you didn't know it consciously. You can now become conscious and sure of this if you try clasping your hands the other way with the other thumb on top, go ahead, try it. . . .
Mrs. B: (*Tries clasping hands differently*) You're right.
Therapist:. . . . and find that it is uncomfortable to clasp your hands that way.

The therapist is again pacing the client's experience by predicting the discomfort of clasping hands in an unusual manner. This successful prediction gains him some credibility with the client, which strengthens the likelihood that she will accept his subsequent leading suggestions. The purpose of the use in the session of the hand-clasping exercise (which is an Ericksonian exercise) is three-fold. First, it begins to redistribute the client's attention away from usual foci of attention that maintain a generalized reality orientation. Second, the suggestions about unconscious knowledge and ability are intended to create a response set, priming or sensitizing the client to the possibility of using natural capacities to follow suggestions for forgetting which are made later. Third, the discussion of unconscious ability points out a view concerning volitional behavior that is a bit different than is usual for the client, and may facilitate the view later that certain cognitive processes can occur automatically and without conscious effort.

Therapist: You didn't know it consciously, that there was one way that was comfortable, but unconsciously you know many things and can do many things and can trust your unconscious capacities. . . . (*Here the therapist lowers his voice tone, slows his rate of speech, increases his eye contact with Mrs. B., and begins to breath in synchrony with her respiration rate*). . . to get you through many experiences and to remember what you need to and to forget what you need to. You can't consciously forget, but we do forget to remember many things, so many things, because forgetting, in itself, is such a common experience, for anyone, but few of us know that we can also learn to remember to forget.

The nonverbal alterations in the therapist's behaviors help to redistribute the client's attention onto the therapist and what he is saying. The alterations can accomplish this because they create slight incongruities which draw attention. The last phrase spoken was a leading or suggestive statement. The difference and similarity between phrases "forget to remember" and "remember to forget" are mildly confusing and help to depotentiate or disrupt usual conscious strategies of thinking. At this point, Mrs. B.'s attention has been distracted from features of the current environment which provide anchors for orienting her to her everyday reality. Her attention is now focused on internal processes. The "early learning" analogy which is used below, a common Ericksonian technique, will also focus her on internal memories, suggesting to her that she can learn to forget, just as she learned to accomplish difficult tasks in the past.

Therapist: And learning new things can be difficult. You may remember back when you first learned your ABC's. Think of how difficult it was to write those letters A (*pause of two seconds*), B (*pause of two seconds*), C (*pause of two seconds*), D (*pause of four or five seconds*), E. . . .

The pauses of two seconds built an expectation that a letter would occur every two seconds. This expectation was then violated to disrupt or depotentiate conscious sets of expectation and thought, creating a subjective sense of being unsure of what to do next. The therapist's next suggestions are intended to lead and restructure the client's experience.

Therapist:. . . . and you discovered that one day you felt (*voice tone drops*) comfortable and relaxed (*voice tone rises*) with your learning experience. . . .

By means of voice tone alteration, a suggestion is interspersed for the client to feel "comfortable and relaxed."

Therapist:. . . . because you could do it, as if it happened by itself, little by little, by natural unconscious processes, without effort, automatically. (*At this point, her eyeblink reflex and respiration rate are slowed, there is no observable bodily movement, her eyes remain fixed on the therapist's, and her facial features are smoothed out due to relaxation.*) And just as you were able to do so in the past. . . .

This last statement is another example of maintaining rapport, or pacing the client's experience, preparatory to a leading suggestion.

Therapist:. . . . you can find yourself, little by little, able to apply new learning to your problem, without effort, and just by listening.

This last sentence suggests that what she is now experiencing and how she will later solve her problem does not require volition and will occur in an effortless fashion. The suggestion facilitates the perception that responses are involuntary.

Therapist: This problem, of your thoughts about an urge versus your thoughts of controlling the urge, this conflict reminds me of a story, an old story, of a dog tied to a post. This poor dog tried so hard to get away, and he pulled and he pulled, but the harder he pulled, the tighter the knot became which held him. Finally, after a great deal of pulling, the poor dog became thoroughly exhausted and simply gave up pulling, and let go. And once he let go, the knot gradually loosened and finally the rope slipped from his neck and he was free of the struggle.

This story suggests that conscious attention at controlling her urge will only serve to maintain or increase her obsession with controlling it. There is a danger here, however, of indirectly suggesting that if she abandons control, then she will act out the urge. Therefore, the next story clarifies that neither the urge nor the control are being abandoned. It is the conflict between them that is abandoned.

Therapist: Like your problem, this problem of the dog tied to the post is similar to the problem of a woman I know who wanted to give up cigarettes. She knew all of the health hazards but this wasn't sufficient reason for her to give up smoking. She had a wish or a desire to control her urge to smoke because she hated to be controlled by this urge. And this urge was strong. She tried to forget the urge, but could not forget it. Then she tried to give in to the urge and forget her desire to control the urge. But she couldn't do this either because she kept thinking she should control her urge. So there she was, in a dilemma, in a conflict between this urge and this need to control it, and she thought about this conflict all day long, every single day. It obsessed her and exhausted her, all the time wishing to give in to the urge and wishing to control it, and knowing that neither wish could win.

These last few statements exactly mirror the client's dilemma.

Therapist: Finally, she became so tormented with always thinking about this conflict that she decided to get rid of all the obsessing once and for all by giving up smoking. She just gave it up, she just dropped it, in order to get rid of the conflict, to forget it, to free her mind. She did not do it for health reasons and she did not do it because she lost the urge. You see, she didn't give up the urge. She gave up the conflict between the urge and controlling the urge. She forgot it and was free. Forgetting is something anyone can do, like forgetting of a dream, or forgetting of an important appointment, or, forgetting the details of a movie when someone asks if you saw it, because it is so easy to do and we have the abilities to do it, but it is difficult to do it consciously. It can be done without conscious effort and is similar to many experiences that we all have. Like when I stub my toe badly when involved in carrying some heavy suitcases, or when involved in listening to a good story, or when involved in some other engrossing activity.

This story of stubbing one's toe will combine the conflict depicted in the two previous stories with more detailed suggestions for forgetting.

Therapist: While I'm engaged in the engrossing activity, I might not even know I've hurt myself until after I've completed the activity. Why did it not hurt? And why does it hurt so much only now? And the pain is something I may try to wish away by conscious effort, but the more you try to wish it away, the more you feel it, and you're caught in a dilemma, a conflict, between wishing it away but feeling it more, and then someone walks into the room and engages you in a conversation and you forget the pain, or a certain thought occurs to you which leads to another thought and pretty soon you can be thinking and doing and feeling other things and find that you've forgotten all about the pain.

These were suggestions for her to take opportunities to allow her attention to be distracted from her conflict, to forget it, and to allow this phenomenon to occur on its own.

Therapist: And you can go about your daily life thinking all sorts of things and enjoying different experiences and completing various tasks until suddenly you may notice the pain throbbing in your toe, and then you remember stubbing it, and then you really feel the pain again, and feel surprised also at the natural ability you have to have forgotten about it all this time, and also feel surprised at the inability to consciously wish it away, and this conflict between the feeling and the wish to control it, this conflict can easily be forgotten once again, in the same way as before, by noticing a distracting thought which leads to another thought, and as time goes on you can learn to do it more and more easily, without any effort. And as soon as you really understand that we all have this ability, you might feel pleased about knowing it. Now, you may easily wonder, "Am I supposed to do certain homework to accomplish this forgetting? What should I specifically do to forget my conflict? To forget my obsession? Should I try to forget it?" No, that wouldn't work. Conscious efforts and trying wouldn't work at all. Do not try to forget it. You do not have to try to do anything at all. But if you find yourself irresistably seduced into trying to do something with voluntary effort, then if you wish, you can do something consciously that might trigger the learning of these unconscious processes of forgetting. You can take opportunities, whenever you can, of noticing some pain or ache or itch, noticing certain sensations in your body. And whatever feeling you choose to notice, you can try to consciously wish it away and find that you cannot do so while you are paying attention to it, but then allow a thought or a sound or a feeling or an event to lead you to another thought and distract you into forgetting what you had been doing.

The therapist has now given Mrs. B.'s conscious attentional processes something on which to focus as a distraction, so that she does not have to feel compelled to try to consciously forget the conflict, which might interfere with the suggestions for forgetting. This also constitutes a ritual which is within voluntary control and which implicitly conveys the message that by engaging in the ritual, her conflict will be forgotten. Whether this cognitive ritual actually triggers or accesses processes of distraction cannot be known with certainty without empirical testing. The following suggestions elaborate on this if-then causal feature. These are not very indirect suggestions and are more typical of more direct approaches.

Therapist: And you can practice like this on trivial sensations, and you won't have to do anything at all in regard to forgetting your problem. You can practice as little or as much as your attention needs something to do until you find that many other interesting things have come to occupy your attention.

As is evident from the above statements, a clear bi-level message has been conveyed: your obsession will be forgotten, but do not try to directly forget it with conscious effort.

Therapist: Until now your current life, your current concerns, can be thought of as a picture, with your conflict, your obsession, in the foreground of the picture, and everything else in the background. And little by little, as you forget to remember this obsession more and more, other things will begin to occupy the foreground of the picture, the foreground of your attention, until you gradually notice that the obsession is becoming part of the background, little by little, drifting further into the background. And you can begin to notice, with perhaps a pleasant surprise, the periods of time you have forgotten your conflict. Of course, you may notice right away, but then again you may not notice for a few days, or even a week, it is difficult to say when it will be. And when you do, you may begin to wonder why you have forgotten so easily, which may puzzle you, but you can trust at that point that your own abilities are healing you and that somehow it all does make sense and that you don't need to figure anything out and that you don't need to do anything at all and can allow other thoughts to lead to other thoughts and go on with enjoyable everyday experiences and tasks.

The last several lines address the cognitive dissonance which Mrs. B. may experience upon wondering why she is not as obsessed as she used to be, which could cause her to feel unlike herself and motivate her to obsess again in order to feel more like herself.

Therapist: And now that you know what to do. . . .

This tells her that she knows what to do consciously.

Therapist:. . . . really know. . . .

This addresses unconscious knowledge and abilities.

Therapist:. . . . you can tell me some more about that project at work and how you're making out with it. Didn't you tell me there were some real bad snags with that? Maybe it's too much for you. Do you realize the difficulties ahead of you with this project? (*The therapist has begun to shift his tone back to normal, quicken the rhythm of his speech, glance away from Mrs. B.'s eyes, cross his legs and engage in normal bodily movement.*)

The rapid shifts in the therapist's behavior and comments focus attention away from inner experience and onto the current environment. These shifts are equivalent to methods of trance termination in formal uses of hypnosis.

Mrs. B: Yes. I do. I think. (*She quickens respiration rate, increases bodily movements, and glances around the room.*)

Therapist: Maybe it's too much for you. And maybe you won't get enough out of it for all your efforts.

Mrs. B: No, no. It's worth it. But I still have a lot of hard work to do.

Therpaist: Well, good luck with it. (*There is a brief conversation about the project at work. Then the therapist gives Mrs. B. another appointment and she prepares to leave.*)

Mrs. B: (*As she walks towards the door*) Gee, I feel so relaxed. Did you hypnotize me?

Therapist: Sort of.

Mrs. B: (*Laughs*) Well, see you in a couple of weeks.

Due to the therapist being ill, the fifth session occurred a month later. Mrs. B. had been practicing the conscious forgetting technique on trivial matters as directed. Her use of alcohol and medication had entirely ceased. The obsession was now experienced only occasionally and was described as being in the "background of the picture" of her current concerns, while the "foreground" was occupied by other thoughts, such as her work project and moving out of her parents' home. However, the loss of her obsession occasioned feelings of sadness. The therapist discussed this loss with her and helped her to mourn this loss, now that she had really let her lover go.

She was also advised to be alert to a re-emergence of her urges to contact her former lover and to be alert to rationalizations she might employ to act on those urges. Instead, she was to prepare a repertoire of alternative behaviors for those occasions. In this session, some of the suggestions for forgetting which were used in the previous session were repeated.

In the next two sessions, a cognitive restructuring approach was taken to address Mrs. B.'s fear of abandonment, her need to feel more adequate, and her need for approval. She was also helped to continue experimenting with distancing maneuvers in interactions with others. Constructive ways to meet needs which her lover had met were also explored. As she felt stronger and more in control, she was advised to expose herself to contacts with her former lover, since accidental contacts were inevitable, and was helped to experience these contacts in a different way than when she was obsessed.

She was also helped to consider the advantages and difficulties of living on her own relative to living with her parents or with her husband. She finally decided that she wanted to live with her husband again because the two of them had become better companions and marriage to him represented a security and stability which had always been important to her. These advantages were more important to her than her husband's "insensitivity" to her needs and the fact that he did not make her feel "special." She was willing to settle for this compromise, and claimed to feel comfortable with the decision.

Mrs. B. decided to terminate therapy following the seventh session, at which time she felt quite in control of her life once again, having only occasional yearnings for her former lover. Her desire for rapid termination of therapy grew out of a feeling of success, but also out of a fear which she now expressed of becoming too rapidly dependent on the therapist. This surprised the therapist.

It is possible that a dependence had formed more rapidly than the therapist had been aware because he had been so directive and Mrs. B. had been so compliant, and he had, in effect, capitalized on her transference to him. That is, he had failed to take adequate cognizance of the possibility that she had been as eager to please him as she had been to please other men in her life. If he had thought about this earlier, he could have encouraged some disobedience towards himself as a way of addressing this problem more efficiently. He had noticed the transference in the first session because it was his own countertransferential reaction to it that had confirmed for him a hypothesis that had emerged from the history, namely, that Mrs. B.'s typical style with men was to please them in a way that made them feel very important; this hypothesis had even led to some useful interventions.

He probably had not addressed the transference because the presenting problems had frightened him, he had feared failure, and he had felt more secure in maintaining Mrs. B.'s obedience in regard to his directives. By this, he may have done her an inadvertent disservice if the result was a dependence which frightened her out of therapy before she was ready. But, then again, she might have been ready. It was uncertain.

The therapist took the opportunity to discuss some of these considerations with her, those about which it was appropriate to do so, in order that she could consider the possible value of continuing in therapy without an unrealistic fear of becoming dependent on the therapist. Yet, the therapist did not wish to persuade her to stay in therapy for any longer than would be useful for her. In this discussion, Mrs. B. remained highly ambivalent about terminating, yet was leaning towards termination. She seemed to be asking permission to terminate or for advice to remain in therapy, so the therapist gently pointed this out. He nourished her growing independence by encouraging her to terminate if she wished but made it clear that he was available as needed. He also made it clear that it was all right if she was angry at him for not deciding for her (hopefully undoing the previous errors), but that it remained her decision. She decided to terminate.

Several months later, Mrs. B. called the therapist to tell him that her obsession about her lover was returning. On the phone, the therapist utilized selected aspects of suggestions previously made which appeared appropriate to the immediate problem. These suggestions seemed to address the problem to a degree sufficient that Mrs. B. no longer felt a need for an appointment.

Brief phone contacts for similar problems with the original lover and new romantic interests occurred approximately six months and a year following therapy, but appointments never appeared necessary. These phone contacts served the function of "booster shots"; they realigned patterns of Mrs. B.'s cognitive processing which were drifting out of alignment and helped her to maintain her path of positive change. They also served to provide follow-up information which indicated that Mrs. B. had managed to put her lover aside and that she considered herself satisfied in her marriage.

Discussion

Suggestions for forgetting. The word "amnesia" was used earlier at one point because instructions for forgetting were employed. However, since Mrs. B. did not entirely forget her lover or her urges to contact him, her experience of forgetting can be considered only a partial amnesia and perhaps not an amnesia at all according to certain definitions of the word. It was certainly not identical to the more dramatic amnesias and dissociative reactions which are sometimes produced in hypnosis. Mrs. B. remained aware of her obsession, but the obsession took a place in the "background" of her current concerns as was suggested to her.

There was nothing mysterious about the suggestions for forgetting. The intervention primarily addressed cognitive processes associated with attention and distraction. By means of the models provided by the stories, Mrs. B. learned in a brief span of time to allow her attention to be distracted from her obsession and to selectively attend to other perceptions.

Suggestions for forgetting were employed for a few reasons. First, an obsession regarding a lover can be a very difficult problem, is not always responsive to usual treatment approaches, and in some people has lasted for years. Perhaps it is such a difficult problem because conscious efforts to solve it serve instead to maintain it as a problem. The overiding goal of the intervention presented here was to block those conscious efforts.

The suggestions for forgetting were used at a particular stage in Mrs. B.'s therapeutic progress. It is a stage in which an unfortunate behavior has been eliminated from daily activities and other behaviors have replaced it, but in which an obsession about that former behavior begins to dominate the person's thoughts. Obsessions of this kind are also common at a certain stage in the elimination of other problems, such as smoking and drinking.

For example, during the early stages following the decision to quit smoking, the urge to smoke is elicited by numerous habit associations of everyday circumstances. Gradually, as new habits are formed, the urges diminish in frequency and a recognition occurs that the need to smoke no longer exists. Previously, most daily activities and thoughts were related in some way, either directly or indirectly, to smoking, and at this stage they are not. However, at this stage a cognitive obsession sometimes develops about smoking a cigarette, without necessarily being associated with an affect or physical craving. This obsession can lead to giving in to the urge, with the rationalization of ". . . . just to see what it tastes like again," and an eventual resumption of the smoking habit. Therefore, it is a precarious stage in the life of a habit problem. It was judged that Mrs. B. was at a similar obsessional stage when the suggestions for forgetting were employed.

Although stories do not have to be used in hypnosis, they are a common feature in indirect approaches because they are valuable in a variety of ways. Stories were used in this case for three reasons. First, it is often easier for clients to attend to their conflicts or dilemmas when these are distanced and displaced onto someone else, such as characters in a story. Second, stories are inherently dramatic, thereby sustaining interest and trance-like behavior.

Third, suggestions which are couched in stories may be met with less resistance and may have more impact than verbal and logical advice because stories immediately establish multiple linkages to a listener's internal imagery and associational processes. These linkages make it possible to more readily internalize therapeutic aspects of the stories. Because these linkages are numerous and overlapping, they can create a resonant impact. Direct suggestion and verbal advice, on the other hand, are more likely to be processed at primarily a verbal and intellectual level, with the processing subject to the limitations of attentional capacity or short term memory.

Unlike Erickson's usual style of storytelling (Erickson, 1980; Erickson, Rossi, & Rossi, 1976; Rosen, 1982), in which meanings are often obscure and not readily understandable to the client, it can be noted that there was a great deal of direction used in this case to repeatedly link aspects of the stories to aspects of the client's experience. This emphasis on clarity was due to the therapist's belief that Mrs. B. required a high degree of direct guidance (or explicit cognitive models for her cognitive behavior) and does not imply any criticism of more ambiguous and indirect methods of storytelling.

A choice is necessarily made in each case of storytelling about the degree to which the story's suggestions will be vague versus explicit. It is sometimes important to utilize vague metaphors and truisms, sometimes so vague that they are mysterious and confusing. A high degree of ambiguity is desirable when the therapist intends for the client to search for meaning and is uncertain about exactly how and to what extent the story's messages will establish linkages to the client's inner associations. It might also be the therapist's purpose at times to allow the client to make those linkages in his own way and in his own time. The potency of vague, ambiguous, and truistic messages can be appreciated by reflecting on the ability of most people to find personal meaning in a Delphic Oracle, in a fortune cookie, or in an astrological chart. The confusion occasioned by ambiguous messages also conveys the implicit message that some incomprehensible ritual or technique is in progress which will cause change to occur.

On the other hand, it may be preferable for stories to contain instructions and suggestions which are explicit in cases in which there is a danger that the suggestions will be misunderstood or misapplied. This may reflect a more direct than indirect approach to change and is epitomized by the social learning model which assumes that therapeutic change often occurs only after the therapist has persuaded the client of the truth of the therapist's theories, whatever those theories may be. Yet, in effect, this assumption is equivalent to the assumption in strategic and indirect hypnotic approaches that change can occur only after the therapist understands the client's world view well enough to use it to effect change. What is important in either case is the therapist's confidence that a shared view of reality has been established.

The therapist's fear that a shared view had not been adequately established led him to make many suggestions more explicit than is sometimes done, and even to explain to Mrs. B. why some of the interventions would be effective, rather than just employing the interventions without explanation of their rationales. Because the therapist did not have the same faith in the "techniques" of psychotherapy that many other therapists do, he attempted to increase the probability that any given technique would have a positive effect by constructing a reality that would support it. This was done in a hypnotic manner despite the fact that explanation of theoretical rationales have the appearance of directiveness rather than indirection. This will become more apparent in the illustrations in subsequent chapters which utilize methods of hypnotic ritual.

A technique which was attempted in the storytelling was that of creating a resonant impact on Mrs. B. by overlapping three stories with the same theme of conflict between desire and control of the desire. It is impossible to predict the degree to which linkages between stories and clients' internal associations will be meaningful because it is impossible to know which of the concepts and images in a client's associational system are more or less meaningful. If therapeutic aspects of a story establish a linkage with a relatively weak and nonmeaningful concept, the therapeutic impact of the story may be jeopardized by the weakness of this link. This potential hazard can be minimized by repetition of the therapeutic theme, but clothing each repetition in different content. The changing content makes a difference in which concepts and images are accessed in the client. The more linkages that are established, the greater the chances are that a therapeutic suggestion will resonate throughout the associational system, with stronger linkages buttressing weaker ones with redundant information. The more a suggestion resonates throughout an associational system, the more it has become a part of the system.

The storytelling also reflected an attempt to suggest what Watzlawick et al. (1974) would describe as a "change of a change." That is, it attempted to estabish an accelerating momentum in the process of forgetting. The implicit suggestion was that Mrs. B. would not only forget, but would become increasingly familiar with processes of forgetting and better able to facilitate this process. The suggestion for this change of a change was made by creation of a parallel of it in the depiction of momentum in the story content. The conflict and the forgetting of it was first depicted in its barest form in the story of the dog tied to a post. In the successive stories, the process of forgetting was depicted with increasing details, suggesting an accelerating change. It was hoped that if Mrs. B. could feel caught up in the flow of the storytelling that the momentum depicted would be paralleled in her own experience of the process.

Falling out of love. The problem of extricating oneself from a hopeless romantic fantasy or self destructive and anguished relationship to which one feels inextricably bound is a common one, but it is addressed only occasionally in the therapeutic literature. One popular approach, which combines behavioral methods, imagery techniques, and cognitive restructuring, was developed by Phillips and Judd (1978) in a book entitled *Falling Out of Love*. The approach involves a number of interventions, but the central ingredients include the following: "thought-stopping", which interrupts rumination about the ex-lover and allows the building of habits of thinking about nonrelated topics; "silent ridicule," which consists of taking the ex-lover off of a pedestal by focusing on his or her limitations; "positive image building," which meets the need for positive regard that being loved provides and which offsets the poor self concept often occasioned by a lover's rejection; and "systematic desensitization," to address feelings of angry jealousy.

Some of the interventions used in the case described here parallel those described by Phillips and Judd (1978) in terms of their therapeutic purposes. They are part of a package of interventions which have been developed over time which appears to be effective in helping people to extricate themselves from romantic entanglements. They are viewed here primarily as strategic and hypnotic methods but will be identified and discussed interchangeably in terms of other models. They are briefly described below, although an expanded description is being prepared for publication elsewhere.

One major ingredient in this package consists of providing a method for distraction from the lover. In the Phillips-Judd approach, thought-stopping is used for this purpose. In the case illustration, this was accomplished by means of suggestions for forgetting, which fulfilled the hypnotic function of blocking conscious efforts by the client to change.

Redefining the client's view of the lover and reframing the client's urge to contact the lover are also important in most cases. The hypnotic functions of this method were fully described in previous chapters. When the redefinition serves to reduce the importance of the lover, the effect is that of taking the lover off a pedestal, similar to the effect of "silent ridicule." When it is done in a therapeutic setting which is relaxed and in which the client can regard the lover from an unusual perspective (sometimes by means of a time projection into the future), it can help to reduce the client's anger and alter the client's demanding expectations of the lover. These effects may result from desensitization and cognitive restructuring, but the reframing, redefinition, and alteration in world view may be just as relevant. When the client's pursuing behaviors can be reframed as flattering to the lover and demeaning to the client, rather than successful acts of vengeance against the lover, then the client's efforts to refrain from contact have been redefined as effective acts of vengeance. "Getting even" in this way is incompatible with "getting even" by contacts with the lover in the same way that relaxation is incompatible with angry jealousy in the desensitization approach to jealousy; in addition, there is an inherent feeling of control and triumph over the lover which provides an incentive and a reinforcement.

The method of "flooding" is sometimes used in the package as well, in which the client is flooded with stimuli which elicit the problem; in these cases, the stimuli are intended to elicit feelings either of yearning for the lover or anger at the lover. The behavioral rationale for this method is to present these stimuli continuously until they either lose the potency to elicit the problematic feelings or until these feelings undergo fatigue and are replaced by other responses such as boredom.

From an interactional perspective, flooding can be viewed as a paradoxical intervention, as was noted in Chapter Four, because it requests that the client continue to have the problem which the client came to the therapist to eliminate. The client may resist the paradoxical instruction to have the problem by giving up the problem. Also, the client is being asked to have the problem in a different way or under different conditions than usual. This serves to contain and control the problem. It also changes the transactional field in which the problem generally occurs, altering the reinforcement contingencies and the subjective and metaphorical meanings of the problem.

Encouraging the client to become emotionally invested in ongoing projects is another tactic that is often helpful. It is equivalent to the tactic described in previous chapters of establishing a relationship to something other than the problem. It will be recalled that this tactic serves the hypnotic function of blocking self defeating efforts to change and may also constitute a change agent extraneous to the model. Often, these clients' cognitive and emotional lives are dominated by the relationship with the lover in such a way that the relationship has provided the major anchor or orientation for everyday functioning. If this anchor is then taken away, the client may feel not only the effects of loss, but also a sense of disorientation, rootlessness, lack of direction and motivation, and a general anomie.

Since our lives consist of the projects or vocational pursuits which we are at any time currently engaged in, it is crucial that the ex-lover not be the major project in the client's life. If the client cannot cathect to or emotionally invest in any projects, which is sometimes the case, he or she can at least be encouraged to engage in activities which have nothing to do with the lover and which provide new sources of reinforcement. This kind of encouragement, incidentally, is analogous to a behavioral approach to the treatment of depression. The client's emotional investment in a project or engagement in new activities will at least help to occupy the foreground of the client's attention, to some extent replace the obsession and the lover as objects of attention, and provide different incentives and directions for everyday orientation in the world. In the case illustration, these functions were served by Mrs. B.'s involvement in her work project, by her learning more assertive behavior, and by her compliant involvement in exhausting therapeutic tasks.

Cognitive restructuring (Ellis, 1977; Beck, 1967, 1976) and imagery techniques (Lazarus, 1977) are also generally employed to address the client's feelings of low self worth. Usually, the client has made his or her self worth dependent on the approval of others, particularly the lover's approval. It is often useful to explore the client's ultimate fears of abandonment in order to desensitize the client to these fears and to teach the client to keep attributions of self worth as independent of a lover's opinion as possible. In effect these interventions are equivalent to the positive image building of the Phillips-Judd approach. The hypnotic functions fulfilled by cognitive restructuring and imagery techniques have been discussed previously in Chapter Five.

In interactional terms, these clients have generally been pursuers in their relationships with others whereas their lovers have tended to be distancers. This characterization of relationships in terms of pursuing and distancing is one that has been extensively developed by the extended family systems approach (Boszormenyi-Nagy, 1965; Fogarty, 1976), although it is only one type of many complementarities recognized by numerous approaches. The complementary patterns of pursuing and distancing sometimes resemble repetitive dances between individuals in their struggles to titrate an optimal degree of closeness-distance. People who primarily employ pursuit behaviors in their relationships can become victims of a variety of distancing maneuvers, which, due to inexperience with these maneuvers, they do not have available for their own use. Thus, they are locked in a pattern from which they cannot extricate themselves, falling back only on pursuit behaviors in their efforts to solve their problems and feeling as if they can too easily get their "buttons pushed" without being able to do likewise in return.

Teaching these clients about pursuit and distancing patterns can be helpful to them; also, encouragement to experiment with distancing maneuvers in safe contexts aids in liberating them from a constraining interpersonal script. The therapeutic intent is not to teach them to become sociopathic manipulators but rather to make them aware of the possibility of having at their disposal something more than their limited repertoire of pursuit behaviors. The hypnotic functions that this teaching serves are to block efforts by the client to solve problems in usual ways (i.e., by pursuit behaviors) and to convey the implication, by teaching new behavior, that change will occur. The actual teaching or learning constitutes an agent of change which is extraneous to the hypnotic model.

These various interventions cannot be applied with a successful outcome in every case of a client wishing to sever a relationship because the timing may not be right. When clients complain that they wish to stop thinking about or having contact with a lover, they are almost always ambivalent about this, both wanting and not wanting the lover, and that is the problem. If the "not wanting" is less potent than the "wanting," then therapeutic interventions aimed at severing the emotional tie may easily fail, may be wasted (in the sense of being invalidated, in the client's eyes, for future use), and may contribute to the client feeling like a failure and becoming more hopeless than ever about the problem. It is sometimes better to inform the client that he or she is probably not yet "fed up" enough or ready yet to give up this symmetrical entanglement because the disadvantages do not sufficiently outweigh the advantages. That is, the client is not yet sure enough that he or she wishes to give up this problem and needs more time and experience with it to discover whether this is a goal that the therapist should address.

Concluding Remarks

Although not all of these ingredients have been used in each case of a client attempting to sever a romantic tie, most of them have seemed appropriate for use along with some of the methods described by Phillips and Judd. Different constellations of ingredients are emphasized in each case, depending on which appear to be most appropriate. In the case illustrated in this chapter, it is impossible to say which ingredients were the effective ones or which were more effective than others.

The suggestions for forgetting were the most apparently hypnotic methods used, which gives the appearance in this particular case of a "borrowing" of hypnotic methods. Yet, the reframing, cognitive restructuring, teaching of distancing, paradoxical prescription, and other methods also served hypnotic functions despite being associated with behavioral, strategic, extended family systems, and other approaches. A better use of the transference, which is a psychodynamic consideration, may have also served the hypnotic functions of blocking conscious efforts at change and fostering the belief in change.

It may appear to the reader that I am stretching a point at times when I note that particular therapeutic methods derived from nonhypnotic models fulfill hypnotic functions. However, I make these comments on the assumption that I have previously provided support for them. I hope it will become evident in subsequent chapters, if it is not already evident, that various methods can be used to facilitate hypnotic effects, without taking away from that method any inherent therapeutic value extraneous to the hypnotic model. A full description of the ways in which each method is applied to fulfill hypnotic functions is not possible in each case illustration. If a full description were given of each application of "nonhypnotic" methods used in this case, the hypnotic way in which each was applied would be evident. The behavioral method of flooding is a good example of this in the present case because in its actual application (rather than its brief description here) it contained all the elements of an elaborate hypnotic ritual as well as allowing for behavioral and paradoxical effects. These considerations may not yet be fully evident but subsequent chapters will provide further illustration.

8

HYPNOTIC INTERACTION IN CHILD CUSTODY MEDIATION

The application of hypnotic and strategic principles in the mediation of custody and visitation disputes is described in this illustration. These principles are applied in a general mediation procedure that was recently developed in a mental health court unit, in Troy, N.Y., which primarily provides evaluations to courts. Prior to the implementation of the mediation procedure, the evaluations conducted by this unit ordinarily contained specific recommendations for custody and visitation dispositions believed to be in the best interests of children, in conformance with evaluation procedures outlined elsewhere (Hoorwitz, 1982; 1983; 1984). Only on occasion were cases referred by the court or by attorneys for mediation; only on occasion were cases considered by evaluators to be appropriate for mediation; and only on occasion did both parents agree to attempt mediation when routinely asked about this in the course of an evaluation. Therefore, mediation was attempted in less than 5% of the cases referred to the unit.

It was not considered possible to attempt mediation in every case because mediation typically requires a number of sessions and it was not possible to provide this amount of service for the high volume of referrals being received from the courts. One session mediation procedures, with success rates of about 80%, were reputed to exist in California, but in the California courts there is a mandate of joint custody, which was believed to create a different psychological set of expectations in the disputing parties than existed in New York State where no such mandate existed. In the court unit in which the author conducted evaluations, parties generally hoped to win in an adversarial proceeding. They approached the evaluator in much the same way as they approached the judge, attempting to paint themselves in the best possible light and their opponent in the worst. This tended to put the evaluator in the position of deciding what was best for the child, a decision which would be forwarded to the court in the form of a custody or visitation recommendation.

Over the years, the author had not only been engaging in mediation in a traditional sense but had also been noticing that, in an increasing number of cases, during the course of evaluation it became possible to mediate cases successfully in one session. He also noticed that he could not predict in which cases this would happen. He then realized that it may have been presumptuous to have believed in the past that he possessed the relevant knowledge to determine indications and contraindications for mediation and that perhaps it might be successfully employed in a greater number of cases than he had thought possible.

In discussing these possibilities with a colleague, Kevin Donahue, a policy emerged in which parents were to be given an opportunity during the course of each evaluation to arrive at a mutually satisfactory decision with the help of the evaluator in a mediator's role. Only one extra hour was planned for this purpose so that it would still be possible to handle the volume of referrals for evaluation being received (although extra time was provided in some cases as needed). In each appointment for an evaluation, the interview sequence consisted of interviewing first one parent, then the other parent, then the child, and finally a mediation interview with both parents.

This sequence enabled the evaluator to be in the position of providing a standard evaluation and recommendation to the court in the event that the interview with the parents failed to result in an agreement. It was recognized at the outset that the context (of conducting a court referred evaluation) necessarily dictated a distortion of the mediation process as it is usually understood in the field. This context has been described above so that the illustration of a session, below, is understood in perspective and not necessarily considered representative of mediation in general.

To the author's surprise, the agreements achieved exceeded 80% of cases referred. Some of these agreements broke down after the parties left the office, often in response to an attorney's advice which served to polarize the parties again, or in response to an adversarial set of expectations conveyed by players in the court system. The exact figures on broken agreements are not yet available, but plans are underway to influence the other players and systems involved so that they reinforce rather than undermine the mediation process.

Nevertheless, the fact that over 80% of the disputing parents left the office with agreements in hand surprised the author as well as others. When colleagues asked what was being done that was so effective, the reply was that standard mediation procedures were being employed (e.g., those found in Haynes, 1981, and in numerous articles in the journal *Mediation Quarterly*), as well as strategic and hypnotic methods. Colleagues had difficulty imagining strategic and hypnotic methods being employed in a context such as this. A full description of the procedure and the specific interventions is being prepared by the author and Kevin Donohue for publication elsewhere.

However, an aspect of this mediation procedure is highly relevant to the topic of this book. In mediation of numerous cases, the author noticed that the interaction between himself and the parties was following a familiar pattern. He noticed that on a preconscious level he was deliberately following this pattern because it facilitated a change in the direction of agreements and minimized opportunities for parental interaction to move in other nonproductive directions. Certain maneuvers by the parents were met by predictable maneuvers by the author which in turn were met by predictable maneuvers by parents. When parents deviated from the pattern, it seemed that the author employed stock maneuvers to bring them back to the pattern. Explication of these circular sequences of maneuvers revealed the parameters of a hypnotic relationship.

These maneuvers are identified below in an illustration of a typical dialogue in a mediation session. Although the content changes from case to case and the circular sequences go off into various directions of emphasis, the same skeletal series of maneuvers illustrated below characterizes the interaction in most of these cases. A typical case was chosen for illustration, one that was neither simple nor excessively complicated. The transcript picks up at the beginning of the final interview, following previous individual interviews that same afternoon with the child, the mother, and the father.

Transcript

Mediator: I asked you both to sit down here together with me to see if it's possible for you to come to some kind of joint decision. In trying to meet your own and your child's needs, each of you has been trying to beat the other, trying to win at the expense of the other. As you've seen, this has been somewhat self defeating because by trying to win in this way, you've put the power to decide your lives into the hands of strangers, such as myself, or the probation investigator, or the judge. By doing so, you've seen how you risk compromising your own needs by having a stranger decide your fates in a way which may not be best for your child and which you yourselves may not like in the least. In addition, by trying to meet your needs in this way, by one of you winning and the other losing, you spend a great deal of money on attorney's fees, you lose time from work for court appearances which get repeatedly adjourned, you involve your child in a prolonged uncertainty as to his fate, and you end up bitterly hating one another as you both keep swapping punches in this battle.

These comments convey an explicit message that what the parties have been doing to solve a problem has been creating a problem or making the problem worse. The comments implicitly convey the message that they should stop trying to bring about change in their usual ways. The comments also serve to put the court, the judge, the evaluator, and the system as a whole into a position that is symmetrical in relation to the parents as a conflictual unit. Their belief that the system (of the judge) may have more power than they and that they may both end up losers might then establish a belief that a complementary relationship might be established between themselves and the court system, with themselves in the subordinate position. The way to defend against or to defeat this outside threat is to unite together in a complementary relationship with one another.

Mediator: I would like to give you both this last opportunity to find that you can meet your needs to your mutual satisfaction by arriving at an agreement that leaves the power to decide your fates in your hands as two responsible and authoritative parents rather than your both giving up that authority to strangers. You may discover you are able to do this.

These comments convey the message that the parents will change in the direction of each meeting their needs, but not by means of their usual solutions.

Mediator: Do either of you have a suggestion?

At this point each parent is usually unsure of what to suggest or how to behave, so the author often points out various possibilities that might meet the needs of each. He also sometimes explains the meanings of sole and joint custody, and answers questions. This usually engenders a suggestion by one of the parents.

Mr. S: How about if Tommy stays with me during the week and you have him every weekend, and on vacations too.
Mrs. S: Why should I do that? I already have custody of him.
Mr. S: But you work during the week and I don't and. . .
Mrs. S: But you will be working again and. . .
Mr. S: And he gets along with me better. You have nothing but trouble with him. You can't control him anymore and. . .
Mrs. S: I carried him for nine months, and you didn't. You were out every night partying, and you even wanted me to get an abortion when I. . .
Mr. S: You're the one who began running around, not me, and. . .
Mrs. S: Don't bring up that. You know why that happened. If you want to bring up all the filth, then why don't you tell the doctor about the time that I caught you with my niece. Or what about the time. . .

These responses by the parties can be considered symmetrical responses to one another, but complementary responses to the mediator's message that they change. That is, they are responding to the mediator's suggestion to change by engaging in their usual solution of trying to beat one another. It is useful for the mediator to allow some of this conflict to occur so that each can feel that unfinished business has at least been fully articulated. In this way they do not need to hang on to "loose ends" or issues that each feels must be aired. This is a cognitive explanation which attempts to account for why "catharsis" techniques of venting sometimes seem to make things better and yet sometimes seem to make things worse when they only serve to allow opportunities to practice aggressive responses.

It is also useful to allow conflictual exchanges of these kinds to occur to a minimal extent in order for the mediator to have the opportunity to observe them. The mediator can then use these observations to point out and demonstrate to the parties that they repeatedly attempt to beat each other in this game, and that by employing this usual solution they succeed only in failing to meet their needs.

Mediator: You two can continue to fight like this, if you like, like two children who come to their mother for a decision about who has been more unfairly treated, and I know that each of you has a very good case. But if you do continue like this you will end up in court where strangers will make the decision. Or you can act like responsible parents and figure out what is best for your child. As spouses, you can hate each other as much as you like and behave as much like children as you can, in a manner that I can see makes you both surprised and embarrassed at yourselves because this sort of thing brings the worst out of you. But as parents of Tommy, you will always have a relationship with each other, whether you like it or not, and you're stuck with it. You will always have a relationship as parents of this child Tommy, and if you wish to be responsible parents you may as well realize this now and begin to figure out how to communicate in this parental relationship, figuring out what's best for your child and best for yourselves as well, unless you wish strangers to do it for you in a way that may not be best for anyone concerned. After all, what do I or the judge really know of your lives and what is best for you. Yet you put these matters into our hands by trying to beat each other in this problem. I'll be glad to make a recommendation to the court if you ask me to. Someone has to do it. And if I make a mistake, I can live with it. But can you?

These comments convey the message that they should stop trying to change in their usual ways. It is a message equivalent to the message "Stop lifting your arm on purpose" in a hypnotic arm levitation. It blocks a complementary response to the message of "Change" or "Lift your arm."

Mediator: I know it seems nuts to you, but I suggest that each of you figure out what would make the other happy. In doing this, you may find that you take the wind out of the other's sails, that the other no longer has a need to fight you and that you end up meeting your needs anyway and become a winner. Although you look like you're surrendering, you end up a winner. Also, in doing this you might discover that the range of alternatives acceptable to each of you actually overlaps, a discovery that's been hidden from you in your misunderstanding and in your efforts to beat each other. Also, if you try to figure out what the other wants, you both may discover that the other doesn't really want that, for example, full time custody of Tommy with no breaks at all. Sure, each of you could live with it but wouldn't some breaks be appreciated? Or, if you had full custody and prevented visitation, like you might really want to do, your child could grow up to hate you for preventing a relationship with the other parent and then run away to the other parent after all those years of hard work at being a good parent. Why not let the kid find out what kind of person that parent is on his own?

This is a strategic intervention similar to those developed by the MRI group of asking each party to take a one-down position in order to interrupt a circular sequence of one-upmanship maneuvers. These interventions were developed by the MRI group to address problems of those who "attempted to reach accord through opposition." Taking a one-down position constitutes a metacomplementary maneuver of surrender, which enables the person surrendering to maintain the position of defining the relationship. It also is an intervention which conveys the bi-level message once again: it simultaneously conveys the message that change will occur yet conveys the message that change should not be attempted in usual ways.

A therapeutic response that is often interchangeable with this intervention at this point in the sequence of interaction with the parties is that of suggesting ways in which each parent can meet his or her needs and yet behave like a responsible parent both to the child and in relation to the other parent. For example, "If I was you and wanted to meet the need to do. . . . . , then I would. . . . " It can be seen that the first half of the above statement is a pacing of the client's experience and that the second half is a leading suggestion. Pacing and leading are also applied in suggestions of the following type: "If you want to behave like a responsible parent and meet your child's need for. . . . (pacing), then you might consider. . . . (leading), or "By bringing the best out of yourselves in this way as responsible parents (pacing), you have produced a remarkable change in your relationship in the form of an agreement which can continue even after you walk out the door (leading).

Any of the above responses are possible as maneuvers for blocking the parties' futile conflict and maneuvering them into positions in which they make complementary responses to one another in an attempt to find a way to meet each other's needs. They are used again and again each time the parties begin fighting. The dialogue below picks up where it left off.

Mrs. S: Is it that you want more time with Tommy? Or do you really want full custody?
Mr. S: I'd never keep him from you when he wants to see you. I know he needs you and loves you.
Mrs. S: You better know it. He's been with me all these years until you finally decided you wanted to be a father again and came sailing into our lives and caused all. . .
Mediator: Hold on, hold on. Listen to yourself. That's exactly the kind of talk that will put you back in court with ax in hand and at the mercy of a stranger's decision. Do you see that? And do you see that you were doing so fine in asking what he really wants? And just listen to him. He's saying fine things about you. Why don't you just ask him to finish what he was saying about whether he really wants full custody or just more time.

This interruption once again blocked a parent's attempt to change things in usual ways, and suggested that the parent experiment with a complementary way of relating to the other parent.

Mrs. S: Do you really want full custody? And me to be out of the picture?

Mr. S: To tell you the truth, I don't know if I could handle him full time. That's not really what I want. Besides, he needs a mother too. If you were out of the picture, I don't know how it would affect him.

Mediator: You mean that Tommy would probably be depressed. And imagine the confusion of being yanked from one home full time into another home.

Mr. S: That's right. I don't want to do that to him. I just want some say in his life. And some more. . .

Mrs. S: You have a say. You're always having a say.

Mr. S: That's just not true and you know it.

Mediator: I don't know who is right and who is wrong. If you want someone to decide who is right and who is wrong, then ask the judge to do it, or ask me to decide and send a recommendation to the judge. Is that what you want? Or do you want to discover whether you can find some areas of agreement? You were saying (*to Mr. S*) that you wanted some say in his life, and she says you can have it, and you wanted more time. What else were you saying?

This is another therapeutic interruption with the same function noted in the last interruption above.

Mrs. S: That's right. You can have all the say you want. Is that what you want?

Mr. S: Well, yeah, I want some say in his life, I want to know what's going on at school, and some more time with him. To do things with him. Help him with his homework. Talk to his teachers. I really think that I can help him with this school problem. That's why I thought if he stayed with me during the school week. . .

Mrs. S: No. I won't be a weekend mother.

Mediator: What do you mean?

Mrs. S: I don't like the idea of being a weekend mother. I'd feel like I was abandoning him and he'd feel that way too.

Mr. S: But you could have him every weekend. That's prime time. Weren't you complaining that you don't get prime time because I see him on weekends now and you have to work all week and you have to be the heavy with him?

Mrs. S: That's why I want visitation switched to every other weekend, so I can have some prime time too. I used to have alot of weekend time before you came sailing into our lives and I let you have weekends. That was probably my first mistake. Letting you have weekends. That's why I want it switched to every other weekend.

Mr. S: But then I would get him even less than now.

Mrs. S: But I need some prime time too.

Mr. S: But what if you had him every weekend plus all school vacations.

Mediator: That's a lot of time. Do you realize how little time children actually go to school and how much time they're on vacation?

This comment by the mediator was not only intended to make a point, but also was intended to distract the parents from the symmetrical struggle which was brewing in the hope that they could continue a constructive exchange of views.

Mrs. S: I never thought of it that way.

Mediator: You might actually get to see him alot more that way, and in prime time too. Then you'd be the Santa Claus instead of dad and dad would be the heavy.

Mrs. S: Hah. That'd be a switch.

Mr. S: That's not really what I'm after, you know. I want to be the heavy along with her. And we can both have good times with Tommy. I don't want to just be the heavy and I would be if I had him all during school and work time and her just having him on weekends and vacations. I need a break too.

Mrs. S: I don't think I'd like it either. I'd still feel like a weekend mother.

Mediator: Even with all that prime time?

Mrs. S: That's right. Why can't we just leave things the way they are and change visits to every other weekend? He can have him for two weeks in the summer.

Mr. S: That's not enough. Why do you always have to have things your way? You'll never change.

Mrs. S: You're the one who's so stubborn. Why don't you just leave well enough alone and stay out of our lives. If. . .

Mediator: Hold on there. You're both back at each other's throats. Is that the purpose here?

Until the last two exchanges, the couple had been constructively exploring alternative ways to meet their needs. The last exchange was clearly the beginning of a symmetrical escalation, which was interrupted as was done at previous points in the interactional sequence.

Mrs. S: You see (*to mediator*), this is hopeless. We can't solve this.

This response constitutes a symmetrical response, rather than a complementary one, to the mediator's message that change will occur. It is equivalent to the subject's arm remaining down when the hypnotist asks for the arm to levitate. It conveys the message to the mediator that change will not occur. Instead of arguing, the mediator next engages in a meta-complementary maneuver of surrender. He thereby maintains the position of the one defining the relationship and can take credit for the client's responses by predicting the course of events. His agreement that the situation seems hopeless is a pacing maneuver, but any other comments about change are leading maneuvers. They suggest events which fall within the range of what the parents may perceive as even happening now within them and between them. This interrupts the trajectory they are on, making it possible for them to behave differently.

Mediator: You might be right. Maybe it is hopeless. Maybe we're wasting our time here. Perhaps it would be best to see what happens in court. Maybe you just aren't ready yet to decide for yourselves and need to experience whatever the court will do, even if that results in repeated adjournments, or prolonged litigation, because it isn't easy for judges to make decisions sometimes. Maybe you need that time to experience that things can get even worse or better and maybe worse again and better again in different ways before you can really discover that you can communicate in a way that allows you to arrive at agreements. I wonder when you will realize you can do this.

This meta-complementary maneuver, which agrees that change may not be possible, simultaneously indicates that things can get worse and better, and thereby continues to send the message that change will occur. The very last sentence contains an implicit suggestion that positive change can occur; it is implicit because the explicit question asks when they will realize they can change, distracting them from the implicit assumption that they can change.

Mr. S: I think we can do it now. I'm ready.
Mediator: You think so? Do you too? (*to Mrs. S.*)
Mrs. S: Yes, Probably.
Mediator: What do you suggest?
Mr. S: Well, I don't know. I'm at my wits end.
Mrs. S: Me too.
Mediator: Would you like a suggestion?
Mr. S: Please.

When a creative impasse occurs, it is sometimes useful to provide suggestions for possible agreements, as the mediator does here.

Mediator: Well, it seems you've both essentially agreed to have joint custody and. . .

The mediator here outlines areas of agreement between them in how their needs can be met and also the areas of disagreement. He then suggests that the father have the child every weekend and all school holidays and that the mother have the child during the school week so that she wouldn't feel like a weekend mother.

Mr. S: That's fine with me, I guess.

Mrs. S: It is? That's what you want? You still wouldn't try to get full custody?

Mr. S: No. I could live with that.

Mediator; Are you sure? It's got to be something you really feel you can live with, that you decided on for yourselves.

Mr. S: I'm comfortable with it. I can live with it.

Mediator: But what about you (*to Mrs. S.*) Are you comfortable with it?

Mrs. S: I think so. I'm not sure.

Mediator: You think so? Are you sure you're comfortable with Tommy being with him during the summer? And with you not having any prime time during the school year?

Mrs. S: That's right. I can't go along with that. It just makes things worse. Why do you always have to get your way with everything (*to Mr. S*)? You almost had me snowed just now. I'm going to get railroaded here. This isn't getting us anywheres.

Mr. S: Why can't you be reasonable for a change instead of flying off the handle all the time.

Mrs. S: I have a right to fly off the handle when I'm about to be bamboozled like this. It's just the way you conned me in the divorce agreement.

Mr. S: Conned you. Hah, I'm the one who got the raw end of that deal.

Mediator: Hold on both of you. You get nowhere with this fighting. You can blame me for breaking down what seemed to be an agreement here. I just wanted to point out that you (*Mrs. S.*) might not be able to live with that agreement. But you can maybe figure out something you can live with. It sounds like you're real close.

This is, again, a maneuver to block their symmetrical conflict with one another. As can be seen below, it wasn't successful.

Mrs. S: You're damned right I can't live with it. And I won't. There's just no talking to that man.

Mediator: You don't want to try?

Mrs. S: No. I have trouble even sitting in the same room with him. I don't know how I've been able to do it for so long today. After all the lies and broken promises and cheating, I'll never be able to trust him again.

Mr. S: What about all your lies and the time that you. . .

Mediator: Hold on now. I've heard enough fighting between you to realize it doesn't get you anywhere, except that it gets you both to hurt each other again and again. I do you a disservice by allowing you to swap punches and sling mud at each other like this. If you both are really so intent on getting one-up on the other and winning, then maybe we're wasting our time. You can each take your chances on winning in court if you like. That's the place to take that risk. That's the place to try to beat the other and prove you're right. Not here. Who is right and who is wrong is something I can't know. It isn't relevant to you coming to an agreement if that's what you still wish to do.

This is another attempt to block their struggle with one another. It reminds them that if they persist in a symmetrical struggle with one another that they position themselves as a unit in a symmetrical relationship to a powerful but blind justice system which could wreak havoc in their lives. It motivates them to interact with one another in more complementary ways.

Mr. S: And if we go to court we both may end up not getting what we want. You made that clear enough. How about if she gets every other weekend with Tommy during the school year instead of me getting every weekend. And she would have him during the school year and I'd have him on summer vacation.
Mrs. S: But what about the summer? I can't go all summer without seeing him.
Mr. S: Of course not. You could see him. As much as you want. Every week if you want.
Mrs. S: How about every other weekend, like during the year.
Mr. S: That's fine with me, except when we go away for a couple of weeks on vacation.
Mediator: Sounds to me like your coming to some kind of plan here that meets both your needs as well as Tommy's. I guess when you are at your best as responsible parents you both end up pretty able to work things out with each other. (*To Mrs. S*) How is it sounding to you?
Mrs. S: It's sounding better.
Mr. S: But you know, that means that I don't get to see Tommy for two weeks at a time during the school year. That's an awful long time. He's gotten used to seeing me every week.
Mediator: That's an interesting dilemma, especially since you both seem to be discovering that you can arrive at agreements that feel comfortable to each of you. Why don't you (*to Mrs. S*) think about what might meet his needs and Tommy's needs for some contact during that two week stretch.
Mrs. S: You can phone him. Or better yet, why not visit him on a school night in the weeks you don't have him.
Mediator: On a flexible basis? Or as a routine schedule?
Mrs. S. Well, I don't think he can know yet because he's not working yet, but it's not a problem.

The session continued, with a few more outbreaks of symmetrical conflict between Mr. and Mrs. S. and with blocking maneuvers by the mediator. They finally agreed to joint custody, with Tommy's physical residence with the mother during the school year, physical residence with the father on all school vacations including summer vacation, visitation with each parent every other weekend throughout the year with a weekday visit on alternate weeks, and with holidays alternating between parents from year to year. Some other issues were also included in the agreement but were not relevant to the purpose of this illustration.

Discussion

In the dialogue above it could be observed that a repetitive sequence occurred, with a couple of variations. In a more lean description, unencumbered by content, the sequence can be described as follows.   The mediator conveys the message that change can occur in the form of each parent finding a way to meet his or her needs. However, the mediator also conveys the message that they should not attempt their usual solutions to bring about this change, that is, that they not try to win at the expense of the other's needs. They are urged to abandon solutions of this kind and attempt to help one another, forming a complementary relationship with one another. They are positioned to relate to one another in this way by the mediator having pointed out that persistence in their usual solutions may result in a failure by both of them to meet their needs. As a conflictual unit they are put into a relationship with a system that could affect both of them adversely; recognition of this can motivate them to unite in a spirit of mutual helpfulness.

The parents may then engage in complementary behavior towards one another. When they do so, they are responding in a manner that surprises them, just as trance behavior surprises a person because it seems unusual or effortless. When they fail to respond to one another in this way and instead slip back into arguing with one another, their relationship to one another can be defined as symmetrical; however, their behavior in response to the mediator is identical to the complementary response of the hypnotic subject who attempts to lift his arm in usual ways, on purpose. That is, they are responding to the mediator's injunction to change by attempting to do so in their usual way of trying to win at the expense of the other. When they do this, the mediator interrupts to tell them to stop trying to win at the expense of the other because they each may lose in this way. Each time the mediator interrupts to block symmetrical conflict between the parents, he may do a number of things, such as pacing and leading, modeling, suggesting a one-down approach, or engaging in any of the other maneuvers described in the transcript commentary or the mediation literature.

If the parents persist in their struggle with one another, the mediator interrupts again with the same blocking maneuver. If they respond to one another in a complementary fashion, or at least in a symmetrical fashion in which they politely test one another's limits, interruption is unnecessary except to provide fresh ideas. Whenever they slip back into a resumption of their symmetrical struggle, the mediator interrupts in the same way described above.

As the cycle repeats itself, there may be times when the mediator's interruptions may not succeed in bringing the parents back to complementary exchanges with one another. The parents may instead insist on trying to change in their usual ways, that is, by winning at the other's expense. The mediator can let them know that they are free to attempt to change in this way, but to do so in court, where they may incur certain risks and disadvantages. They are free to make this choice, to exit from the mediation process, and to take their chances. The mediator must respect the parents' rights enough that he or she is prepared to terminate at any instant in order for this maneuver to have the most likely chance of positive effect. If the parents do not leave, they are positioned once again for complementary exchanges with one another.

As the cycle continues to repeat itself, another variation may occur. One or both parents may insist that the problem is unresolvable and cannot change without one winning and the other losing. This is not an attempt to solve the problem in usual ways, but is, instead, a symmetrical response to the mediator's injunction to change. The mediator can meet this response by a metacomplementary maneuver of agreement or surrender, saying, for example, that it seems that perhaps they are not yet ready for change and that things might change for the worse before they change for the better, or wondering when they will realize they are ready. If the parents do not leave, they are positioned once again for complementary exchanges with one another.

Concluding Remarks

On occasion a parent does exercise the right to have his or her day in court. The mediator must be careful not to interfere with this right by manipulation and subtle persuasion that could constitute coercion. The mediator cannot know what is really best in the end and can only provide an optimal interpersonal context for change in the direction of an agreement. An agreement may not be the best disposition for the child and a failure to help parents to arrive at an agreement may well be a fortunate failure. For example, in one case a father broke an agreement that had been achieved near the end of an exhausting session because he believed that the agreement would compromise his child's needs. He was convinced that this was so and was willing to take his chances in court. In this case the mediator might have had a contrary opinion but could not presume to be certain that the father was incorrect. The father may have done what was best in the end although he took risks for both himself and his child by leaving the decision to a court.

An example of another case punctuates that failures are not necessarily poor outcomes. After helping the parents to arrive at an agreement, it was the mediator who stepped out of his mediator's role and back into his evaluator's role to say that he could not condone the agreement. In his role as an evaluator and an expert on children he had to protect the child's interests and could not in good conscience facilitate an agreement that he believed would significantly thwart the child's needs. He apologized for spoiling the agreement but asked them to try again.

There is certainly much more to mediation than is described in this chapter. This chapter is intended only to illustrate a repetitive sequence of maneuvers in the interaction between parents and mediator that seems to facilitate change in the direction of agreements. It is a peculiar sequence of communications that is identical to those evident in a hypnotic relationship. The author believed that to explicate this sequence of interactions in this way might be of some use to mediators and might be of some interest to theorists in the fields of hypnotic and strategic therapy.

9

HYPNOTIC RITUAL FOR THE REMOVAL OF HEADACHE IN A NATURAL SETTING

This chapter illustrates the application of hypnotic methods in a natural setting for the purpose of removing a headache. The ways in which hypnotic methods were applied were somewhat different than in previous illustrations which have been taken from therapeutic settings. These differences in application were dictated by the nonclinical context; their depiction here serves to highlight the diversity of uses and the flexibility of application of hypnotic methods which are possible.

In this case there was a heavy reliance on ritual to bring about a hypnotic or curative effect. Ritual may appear to be downplayed in indirect hypnotic approaches but this is only because these approaches avoid rituals which have rigid forms, especially rituals which are authoritative and which convey the idea that hypnosis is a mysterious state. Rituals are frequently created and used by practitioners of indirect approaches with a flexibility and subtlety that often obscures the fact that they are rituals. Inherent in ritual is the characteristic of incomprehensibility, or mystery, or unpredictability; and this characteristic can play a powerful role in effecting change (O'Connor & Hoorwitz, 1984; O'Connor, 1985). The case example shows how the mystery inherent in ritual can be effectively utilized in an everyday fashion in a mundane context. Before beginning the case example, a few words are said below about the general use of ritual.

Use of Ritual

There was a practitioner in Europe who became known as a famous wart doctor due to his success in curing warts; he did so by painting the warts with bright colors and by turning on an impressive-looking machine which the patient was led to believe had a curative effect. Witches have long been known to have removed warts, headaches, and other ills by chanting incomprehensible incantations, burying assorted ingredients at crossroads, and using other odd rituals. Wise grandmothers who understand the power of ritual have commonly removed the pain of a bruise or solved other problems by extemporaneously creating a ritual for a child to perform, such as turning around three times and holding a finger on one's nose for a minute. The exact content of the ritual is irrelevant as long as it involves a sequence of steps sufficient to distract the child and which the child believes to be efficacious.

The list of examples can go on to include hypnotic applications, therapeutic methods, religious and shamanic uses, as well as applications of ritual practiced in everyday life by lay persons. In all of these examples, a message is conveyed that if a certain ritual is performed, then it will cause a certain curative effect. This message is hypnotic in the sense that the relationship between the ritual and the curative effect involves an "if-then" causal link which is often questionable. It is equivalent to any hypnotic statement of the following form: "If you count each breath you take, then you will soon feel more relaxed and find that your eyelids are becoming heavier." In examples such as this, the presumed cause of the hypnotic effect is not always recognizable as a ritual. In the examples cited earlier (for example, of a witch's incantations), the presumed causes are more obviously ritualistic in the ways they are communicated.

To the degree that the ritual has validity or makes sense within the belief system of the subject, such as appearing to have scientific, medical, or religious validity, or validity in some other respect, a belief in the efficacy of the ritual is enhanced. This belief increases the probability that the curative or hypnotic response will occur. To the degree that the ritual involves unpredictability, incomprehensibility, mystery, or confusion, it contributes to depotentiation of conscious sets or distraction of attention from the question of whether the ritual does indeed contain an efficacious ingredient. This depotentiation and distraction renders the subject more tractable to leading suggestions and also allows time for the subject's cognitive, autonomic, and other internal processes to respond to the suggestions. The characteristic of mystery or incomprehensibility may also engender awe and respect, which can facilitate belief in the effectiveness of the ritual. Therefore, use of rituals may be most effective when they appear to be both valid and incomprehensible.

While hypnotic ritual can be found in probably every application of hypnotic methods in this book, its use is often obscured by other features; in contrast, the use of ritual stands out in bold relief in the case example of this chapter. The characteristic of incomprehensibility is inherent in the ritualistic procedure illustrated here, just as it is in the practices of the wart doctor or the witch. Yet, a ritualistic approach was applied without the fanfare and seriousness that the wart doctor or witch might use and in a more mundane and natural fashion.

A Natural Setting

This case example is included in the book not only because it illustrates the way in which the therapeutic potential of ritual can be maximized but also because it is taken from events which occurred in a nontherapeutic or natural setting. Although the goal was therapeutic, the traditional trappings of therapy were absent and the application of hypnotic methods took on forms unlike those illustrated in other chapters. The case is also of interest because it represents a common event for therapists who are asked by friends or family members to be put in a trance or to be helped in other ways for emergency treatment. Each request of this kind is different and tends to be handled differently by different therapists. Therefore, general rationales are not provided here for when and how therapists should respond or not respond to such requests. Only the author's own rationales in this particular case are provided where they appear relevant.

Since the hypnotic interaction occurred in a natural setting and involved the author, it would be more awkward than it usually is to refer to the hypnotized person as either a client or a subject and to the hypnotizing person as the hypnotist, the therapist, or the author. Therefore, these styles are dropped from this particular case illustration and instead I will describe how I hypnotized Lyman.

Case Illustration: The Removal of a Headache

At the time of this application of hypnotic methods, Lyman was a 32 year old female and a close personal friend of mine. The application occurred in a home setting on an evening in which Lyman experienced an attack of headache that she found close to intolerable. She generally suffered from what she described as tension headaches but this particular headache was causing more distress than usual and she wondered whether it was a migraine. She had asked me numerous times in the past to hypnotize her for various purposes, but I had done so on only one occasion six months earlier. I remarked that I probably should teach her self hypnosis so that she would be better prepared to handle headaches when they came upon her. My thought was to teach her to use hypnosis on some other occasion, in a relaxed and unpressured context, not to utilize it in response to this crisis situation. However, she requested that I utilize it immediately. I wheedled out of it by saying that I was too tired.

Although it was true that I was tired, this excuse was a rationalization. My reluctance was due to other reasons. First, Lyman and I had had a number of discussions about hypnosis in which I had explained how various hypnotic rituals and techniques were used to facilitate hypnotic effects. These explanations had allowed her to see with clarity the dubious logic inherent in hypnotic suggestions. She had poked fun at the dubious cause-effect links between hypnotic methods and hypnotic effects, and this had nourished a skeptical attitude concerning the efficacy of hypnotic methods. She frequently alluded to therapists as "quacks" while at the same time recognizing that some were quite effective.

If I were to use rituals or methods I commonly used, she was very likely to recognize them as topics of conversations we had had. Her recognition of these methods could focus her attention on the question of whether they could cause hypnotic effects, rather than allowing herself to be distracted from these methods to a degree sufficient for hypnotic effects to occur. Since she was also familiar with many of the maneuvers I used in therapy to distract clients from hypnotic methods, she was sensitized and alert to many of the maneuvers I might use with her, to a degree which would have made it difficult for me to stay ahead of her or take her by surprise.

The reasons for my reluctance can be summarized by saying that I feared she would respond with symmetrical maneuvers to my attempts to induce a trance. These maneuvers might only consist of humorous remarks or skeptical thoughts, rather than deliberate attempts to resist me, but they would effectively one-up me and prevent the establishment of a hypnotic relationship. I was unsure I was skillful enough to prevent her from defining the relationship between us as symmetrical. My uncertainty was due not only to her familiarity with my methods and her skeptical attitude, but also to the fact that we had a personal relationship in which she had demonstrated her interpersonal skill by one-upping me with great frequency and exquisite subtlety. Whether or not the therapist can maintain the position as the one who defines the relationship can often account for induction failures and is a worthy issue of concern when a therapist is in the process of deciding whether to attempt a hypnotic induction with any given person.

I was reluctant to risk my credibility as a skilled therapist by attempting a formal trance induction, preferring to use any credibility I had in her eyes in a more advantageous fashion. Formal inductions are necessarily accompanied by some degree of fanfare that conveys the message: "Here comes hypnosis." It may be an implicit message, but it is nevertheless a clear one, suggesting that now we must all stop whatever we are doing to engage in a set of special hypnotic procedures which will have definite effects. The inconvenience and trouble of a formal trance induction can sometimes constitute a lot more hoopla than the result is worth. The possibility of this in the present instance could have created a challenging and exhausting encounter, which might have also become rather tedious and time consuming. In view of the significant doubts I had about effecting a successful outcome, I judged the costs of attempting a formal induction to heavily outweigh the advantages.

I decided to apply hypnotic methods in an informal and unobtrusive fashion, but I did not think that it would be wise to do such things as slow my speech rhythm, lower my voice tone, tell paradoxical stories, and so on, because Lyman had read about these things in previous chapters in which they have been described and illustrated. Therefore, she would be more likely than others to recognize such maneuvers, and judge them to be artificial and manipulative and to wonder whether they would work, despite my best attempts at subtlety.

While trying to think of unobtrusive ways to redistribute Lyman's attention and to apply other hypnotic methods, the idea of handwarming occurred to me. Handwarming is a method that has been used for the treatment of migraine headache due to a theoretical presumption that the dilation and constriction of peripheral blood vessels in the hands parallel relevant vasculature in the cephalic region. This presumption is derived from one of two competing theories about the cause of migraine. The theory proposes that migraine is the result of extracranial vasodilation, which is presumed to be associated with increased sympathetic activity and with constriction of peripheral blood vessels. Therefore, dilation of the peripheral blood vessels by handwarming is assumed to reduce extracranial vasodilation of the temporal arteries. The exact mechanism by which this nervous system mediation is presumed to occur is unknown.

Whether handwarming does in fact cause a reduction in migraine is controversial (Andreychuck & Scrover, 1975; Elmore, 1979; Fahrian, 1977; Mullinex et al., 1978; Sargent et al., 1973), a controversy I had discussed with Lyman in the past. Also, whether handwarming could cause a reduction in tension headaches as well as migraine is also questionable. Yet, Lyman tended to attribute validity to "natural" healing approaches and the idea of handwarming had the aura or flavor of a natural approach. Also, I judged that the rationale for it would sound plausible enough, even scientific, and that handwarming could comprise or could be crafted into the kind of ritual I needed to facilitate a hypnotic response.

The Intervention

I then told Lyman that I knew of something that might help her with her headache and reminded her of the handwarming method and its controversial rationale. I said that if she wanted to try an experiment, that it might be worth putting her hands under warm water for awhile. She said she was ready to try anything at that point, so I told her to turn on the water in the kitchen sink. She stopped what she was doing and readily followed this instruction. Although I was occupied in another activity, I left it to walk over to the sink. I then explained to her again, but in more detail, the biological rationale for the handwarming technique.

I finished my complicated explanation by offering the simple suggestion that the handwarming was likely to work if she just concentrated on perceiving the sensation of warmth. Then I quickly walked back to a task in which I had been formerly engaged in order not to appear as if I was personally invested in the question of whether or not the handwarming technique would work. About a minute later, she turned and asked if she had left her hands under the water long enough. I laughed and jokingly asked her if she was getting bored, which was intended as a way of pacing her behavior. I also asked if the headache pain had diminished at all, to which she replied that it was slightly better. I walked over to the sink, looked at her hands, and told her that what was happening looked good but that the blood vessels could become even more pronounced. I turned the water to a warmer temperature and told her to leave her hands under it for another couple of minutes.

The implicit suggestion was that her headache would diminish as her blood vessels became more pronounced. Also implicit was the instruction to watch the blood vessels for signs of change, an activity which would serve the function of distracting her a bit from the therapeutic suggestion concerning diminished pain. I walked away again, leaving her at the sink where she stared fixedly at her hands. When I returned, her blood vessels were quite visible and she announced that her headache was considerably diminished though still present. Specifically, it was now absent behind one of her eyes and somewhat reduced behind the other.

Up to this point, only suggestions Lyman was sure to follow had been given. Each time she followed a suggestion made it more likely that she would follow subsequent suggestions. Suggestions were given rather sparingly in order to gradually and unnoticeably shape the relationship, temporarily, into a hypnotic one. By this point, a hypnotic relationship had developed and I now felt more free to proceed with procedures which Lyman may have found more questionable at an earlier point. Also, at this point, her attention was distracted from the chores, the topics of conversation, and other activities in which she had been previously engaged. She appeared focused entirely on her perceptions of her blood vessels, on my explanation and observations, on her internal judgements about the degree of pain she still experienced, and probably on a sense of wonder or doubt concerning the fact that the pain had diminished as much as it had. She looked as if she had just been interrupted or woken up from a nap and wasn't sure what to do next. Therefore, I concluded that her attention was redistributed to some extent and that conscious sets were depotentiated. That is, she was poised to be led by further suggestion.

At that point, I said to her that it was good that her headache was diminished and how interesting and puzzling it was that a pain could go away so easily. These statements were intended to pace or mirror her current experience. However, I then told her that there was more to be done after we had gotten the headache down further. This was a comment that avoided a direct suggestion since it contained only an implication or indirect suggestion that her pain would continue to subside as a result of whatever unspecified activity we were about to do, so that afterwards we could engage in some other unspecified activity.

I then took her hands from the sink and told her to stand still for a minute and to just let her body learn how it felt to be without pain, which again implied continued pain reduction. Then I put her hands under the water again for about a minute and then once again removed them, as if I was now following some ritual or some sequence of procedures which I knew to be effective for such problems. I then told her that she had to let her body get used to feeling less head pain, without the benefit of warm water and that we could trick her body into being without that pain.

In the meantime, I told her, the pain that was still present might be handled by sending competing neurological signals to her brain which would block or interfere with signals causing the perception of pain. I then began to supply those competing signals by massaging her head and neck. This massage rapidly distracted her from the suggestion that her pain would continue to diminish and also from the suggestions that her body could learn to feel pain-free in the absence of warm water. The distraction was intended to facilitate an uncritical acceptance of those suggestions and to allow internal and autonomic processes to respond to them.

As I began to massage her, I once again began to provide technical explanations derived from various theories on the perception of pain in order to lend validity to what I was doing and to the suggestions I was making. The semantic content was not crucial to my intentions except insofar as it established validity for the procedures I was applying. This monologue was intended to be somewhat boring and it was not necessary for Lyman to follow every point.

I also interspersed comments, in a less boring tone, which repeatedly conveyed the simple message that pain is perceived or registered in the brain, not in various other sites on the body, and that a pinch or sensation from somewhere other than the source of painful stimulation could block the neural pathways to the brain which conveyed signals of pain. I drove this point home by reminding her of a story I had previously told her about how my dentist had masked the pain of an injection of novocaine by wiggling and stimulating my cheek and lip. I also punctuated these suggestions by occasional pokes and squeezes and rubs which were different from usual massage techniques, which served a distracting function and which appeared to her to send competing neural impulses.

During the massage, I checked with her twice on the location of the pain and on the progress of the pain reduction, which by implication rather than direct suggestion again suggested progress in pain reduction. In doing so, I looked at her with scrunched-up eyebrows in a quizzical, knowing, diagnostic look which suggested that I knew exactly what I was doing, and responded to her answers by massaging what appeared to her to be special places on her head. The first special place met with no effect, so I responded by saying "Aha," as if her response was one possible expected response in this procedure. I repeated my inquiry as to the location of the pain, and when told it was behind the left eye, I said, in a knowledgeable tone of voice, "Ah, no wonder. I didn't realize it was that one."

Then I put my fingers immediately to her neck as if that was the appropriate spot for that sort of problem. This seemed to have a soothing effect. After about two minutes of massage, I asked if she had any further pain. She replied that it was extremely slight and not a problem at all.

I stopped massaging her and told her to just stand there and move her body very slowly, in slow motion, again telling her we had to trick her body into getting used to being without pain in a context in which she was neither warming her hands nor getting massaged. After a minute I again massaged her head briefly for distraction purposes and then stopped and told her to continue to let her body be tricked. When asked how she felt, she said she felt great. However, I told her there was still more to do, in order to generalize this pain-free state to other kinds of activities. I then asked if she was ready for the next step. She looked expectant, laughed, and said yes.

I then pulled her by the hand and ran through the house with her, dragging her down the halls and telling her to go faster all the way. When we arrived at the opposite end of the house, I stopped and massaged her head briefly again. At this point, she appeared thoroughly confused as to my purposes and quite distracted from her pain. I again told her we were still engaged in tricking her body into not having that headache. At that point she said there was only a "smudge" of the headache remaining. I told her that was fine but that we were not yet done. Instead of running back through the house, we had to walk, in order to get her body used to all kinds of normal movements without pain, and that when we were done, it would be sufficient.

We walked back slowly and began to talk about chores and other everyday topics. This served to terminate the intervention as well as to continue to generalize the pain-free state to nonhypnotic conditions. By the time we had reached the other end of the house, we were both walking, talking, and otherwise behaving normally once again and we both went back to activities in which we had been engaged prior to the intervention.

As we did so, she thanked me for getting rid of her headache, saying there was only a "whisper" of it left. She asked if I had put her in a trance, and I responded by saying that I had applied some hypnotic methods and that she may very well have been in a trance. She laughed and said that she didn't doubt it because she had felt she was "going blank'' and ''trancing out'' about the time I began talking about theories of pain, a monologue which she said she could barely recall. She believed she had developed an amnesia for this as well as some other portions of the intervention. But she wasn't complaining. She was quite happy to be pain-free.

I urged her to see a physician about her headaches and she later learned that the headaches were most likely due to either bruxism or TMJ. About a year later, she asked for help with another attack of headache, again in a natural, everyday setting; since warm water was not available, I used massage and some other activities to facilitate pain reduction. Although the content of the activities was different than in the intervention illustrated here, the application of principles was identical.

Discussion

As mentioned in the introduction of this chapter, an interesting feature of this case is the unusual form in which hypnotic methods were applied. This form was dictated by the nontherapeutic context and by Lyman's familiarity with my usual repertoire of hypnotic maneuvers. Fixation of attention was accomplished by directing Lyman's attention to the progress of her blood vessels, rather than by a soothing tone of voice or other more common methods. Pacing and leading statements did not contain recognizable hypnotic content, such as ''As you listen to my voice, you will find yourself discovering something new.'' Instead, the content was unobtrusive and was couched in blunt, everyday language, such as ''It's good that your headache feels a bit better (pacing), but it's not enough (leading).'' Also, many leading suggestions were indirectly communicated by implication from other kinds of statements and behaviors, as was repeatedly highlighted in the case description.

It is possible that handwarming or the head massage, singly or in combination, were effective ingredients in diminishing the pain. However, because these methods have frequently been ineffective for headache, I did not want to have to count on them. I regarded them as methods that might possibly help, that wouldn't hurt, and, more importantly, that could be used to craft a ritualistic experience which would produce a hypnotic effect. They lent validity to the ritualistic experience and helped to foster a belief in its efficacy.

It should be obvious, however, that the ritual consisted of more than either handwarming or massage. It consisted of the entire experience, beginning with the turning on of the faucet and ending with the leisurely return from the other end of the house. One of its distinguishing features as a ritual was the use of rapid transitions from one activity to another, for example, going from handwarming to massage and then back to handwarming and then running, then massaging, and finally walking. This was done as if the particular sequence of activities mattered in regard to the efficacy of the entire procedure, but in a way that was intended to appear perfectly comprehensible to me and somewhat incomprehensible to Lyman.

The incomprehensibility and unpredictability of the sequence of activities produced depotentiating effects which rendered Lyman extremely responsive to leading suggestions. More importantly, they distracted her from her headache, resulting in her noticing, subsequently, that her headache bothered her less. They also distracted her from suggestions indicating that her headache would diminish, allowing time for her expectations and beliefs to mobilize autonomic processes that would actually reduce the pain.

The amnesia, or incomplete memory for parts of the experience, is typical of trance, even trance which is unexpected. It may be due to attentional absorption or distraction, which may create a sense of disorientation and interrupt the usual habits of information processing. In this way the organization and storage of incoming information may be affected, as well as the retrievability of that information.

The question can be raised as to whether Lyman's subjective perception of "going blank" is crucial to defining the experience as a trance. If that subjective perception had not occurred, should the entire experience be considered to be nothing more than the effects of misdirection, similar to the effects achieved by parlor magicians, illusionists, or prestidigitators? While the "going blank" rendered the experience more exotic and more recognizable as hypnotic, I do not think it is necessary in defining the experience as trance. The "going blank" was probably a result of the degree of attentional distraction which happened to exist in this situation, a degree which is not necessary to all trances nor to all points in a trance. Whether or not Lyman realized trance had occurred was independent of the fact that her headache had been diminished by the application of various hypnotic methods.

More important than whether or not a person recognizes that trance is occurring is the person's perception that responses are involuntary. When a therapist suggests that an arm will levitate, or that a headache will diminish, or that an obsession will be forgotten, the therapist does not want the person to attempt to follow the suggestion with conscious effort or to conclude, after the hypnotic response occurs, that it occurred by an act of conscious effort, for example, that the subject lifted his arm on purpose in order to be compliant. In the case of headaches, obsessions, and many other clinical problems, the client cannot get rid of the problem by compliance or by conscious effort; that is why the client is asking the therapist for help. Conscious efforts to get rid of the problem have already been applied and have probably been maintaining the problem. They also serve to lock the person into a symmetrical struggle with the problem. Therefore, the therapist does not say, "Snap out of it and get rid of your headache." Instead, the therapist must be able to convey the bi-level message, "Get rid of your headache but do not do so on purpose."

As was illustrated in this chapter, the hypnotic or curative response can be facilitated by fostering the belief that certain acts or rituals, if properly performed, will cause the response to occur on its own. Whether these are exotic rituals or simple instructions to listen to the therapist's voice does not matter as long as the person believes they are effective. The therapist may also use knowledge of behavioral science or other sciences (e.g., handwarming, behavioral principles of "response generalization," or theories about pain perception) to arrange conditions likely to produce the curative or hypnotic effect, but may distract the client from these conditions in order to facilitate the perception that the effect is occurring on its own and without the kind of conscious struggle which might interfere with the effect. Whatever the actual cause for the diminution of the problem, an optimal context for change is created by the client giving up conscious efforts to change, or taking the stance that change will occur on its own. This client stance depends on the therapist maintaining the position of defining the relationship so that he can effectively convey the paradoxical message that the client should get rid of the problem but should not do so on purpose.

Concluding Remarks

Ordinarily, "hypnosis," with all its trappings, myths, and distracting rituals, creates an ideal context for a therapist to convey the message that the client should get rid of symptoms but should not try to do so on purpose. However, this message is conveyed in nonhypnotic contexts as well, as this and previous chapters have illustrated, with the client engaging in certain behaviors or rituals with the expectation that those behaviors will cause curative effects to occur on their own. As previous chapters have shown, this message is usually conveyed with subtlety and in disguised forms, with the result that the use of ritual or of hypnotic methods is obscured. That is, the presumed causes for the hypnotic effects do not ordinarily take on specific forms which are recognizable as rituals or as "hypnotic."

In the present case, I thought it necessary to give the presumed cause for the curative effect a specific form which had the obvious appearance of an incomprehensible but valid ritual. The characteristics of incomprehensibility and validity were necessary to rivet and distract Lyman's attention and to foster the belief that the headache would diminish on its own without her conscious effort. The use of ritual gave Lyman something to do that she believed would cause change and helped to push the headache from the foreground of her awareness, where conscious efforts to handle the problem were probably helping to maintain it. It also provided me with a tool to establish a hypnotic relationship with Lyman. This altered her conflictual, symmetrical relationship to the symptom, repositioning her in such a way that the symptom could appear to be less potent, less troublesome, and to go away almost as if it were doing so on its own.

10

EXORCISM OF VOICES WITH A HYPNOTIC AND STRATEGIC USE OF RITUAL IN FAMILY THERAPY

Hypnotic methods were used in the case presented here to address the problems of auditory hallucinations and suicidal behavior in a child. The parents were present during the intervention and played roles which were choreographed to serve specific strategic functions. The intervention consisted of a combination of hypnotic methods and certain of the strategic interventions described by Madanes (1981). These and their theoretical rationales will be discussed following the case presentation.

Case Example: Auditory Hallucinations

Patricia K., the youngest of three daughters, was 12 years old when her parents contacted a mental health agency requesting help for Patricia's auditory hallucinations. She had complained of hearing voices after a short stay at a summer camp which was sponsored by a religious order. She had been exposed there to some discussions and lectures which had frightened her, about death and about good and evil. While there, she had also worried about the health of her family, had become homesick, and had requested that she be allowed to leave the camp. However, the camp director, nicknamed Sledge, had not allowed her to leave. Patricia then became so upset that some camp counselors took it upon themselves to call Mrs. K to inform her of Patricia's condition.

Mrs. K. arrived at the camp a short time later and decided to take Patricia home, despite the director's disapproval. As Patricia and Mrs. K. prepared to leave, Patricia noticed that Sledge, the director, looked angry and disappointed in her. As the car pulled away and as Sledge passed out of view, Patricia was heard to say that Sledge was now in her sleeping bag, which was packed in the trunk of the car. This was the first clear evidence of any magical thinking or disorder of perception.

The problem worsened after Patricia arrived home. She began to complain that she was hearing Sledge's voice telling her that if she did not come with him, then something terrible would happen to her family and to her pets. She also began to refuse to attend school because she complained that the hallucinations occurred in that setting as well. This school refusal was of considerable concern to her parents because Patricia had had academic difficulties the previous year and they feared that she might fail a grade as her two older sisters had. At home, she was anxious and fearful a great deal of the time, feeling safe only in a chair that her father tended to use.

At that point, the family contacted the county mental health agency where a psychiatric evaluation and supportive counseling were provided. Also provided was consultation with school personnel intended to maintain Patricia in the school setting despite her fears. Attempts were also made to help her to feel less anxious at home by expanding gradually the "safe spot" which her father's chair represented. In addition, she was also put on a low dose of Mellaril by the agency psychiatrist.

However, following a month of treatment, the hallucinations persisted and the problem worsened. Patricia began to say that she wanted to kill herself and was even found standing in the middle of a crossroads. The family responded by becoming more protective, attempting to make sure that someone was usually with Patricia. She had also developed severe headaches, for which she was evaluated both by her pediatrician and a neurologist. They found no evidence of migraine or of a neurological problem and one of them suggested that the parents take Patricia to a hypnotist for treatment of her problems. The family did not know whether to remain with the agency, where hypnosis was not being provided, or to seek treatment from a hypnotist.

At this point, due to staff changes, the case was transferred to the agency's psychiatrist, who was asked by the family whether hypnosis could be used. The psychiatrist consulted the author to ask whether hypnosis would be appropriate and, if so, whether the author would provide it. After she had communicated to the author all of the information presented above, the author concluded that the information available did not enable him to understand the nature of the problem well enough to make treatment recommendations, including recommendations for hypnotherapy.

The author did suggest to the psychiatrist that she tell the family that a hypnotist available to the agency had been consulted and that the hypnotist had suggested a better understanding of the problem was required before determining an appropriate treatment plan. He suggested that she also inform the family that they were free to seek help elsewhere if they desired, but if they decided to remain with the agency that the psychiatrist would have to take the time necessary to adequately understand the problem since she was new to the case. She followed this advice and felt less pressured as a result. The family also decided to remain in treatment at the agency rather than seek out a hypnotist.

However, in the following two weeks Patricia's hallucinations and suicidal threats increased to the point that she was hospitalized for reasons of safety. Due to this escalation, the psychiatrist asked the author to accompany her to the hospital in order to meet with Patricia and her parents and to help to intervene if effective intervention seemed possible at this point. Up to this point, the author had hoped to avoid contact with the family in order not to risk undermining the psychiatrist's footing with them. However, it seemed that this was a risk worth taking, since the psychiatrist was clearly asking for direct intervention of some kind.

The Intervention

Evaluation of the problem. When the author and the psychiatrist entered the hospital room and the author was introduced, the author assumed that the family knew that he was the hypnotist that the psychiatrist had told them about. This turned out not to be the case; they did not become aware of his identity until later in the day. Therefore, the author's intervention cannot be considered to have been conducted in the context of a formal trance induction.

The author first greeted Patricia, who sat on her bed looking weepy and woebegone. She was miserable about having to stay in the hospital and wanted to go home. He then turned to the parents, asking them a number of questions and engaging each of them in the process of revealing information which he made clear would help to figure out this problem.

He had previously thought that Patricia's headaches and other symptoms might be metaphorical for headaches and problems her father might be having and therefore be serving a protective function by bringing out the parental best in Mr. K. He found, however, that Mr. K. had no such problems. The author also ruled out any history of similar problems in the family concerning hallucinations, depression, or bizarre behavior.

He was able to confirm an observation made by the psychiatrist that Mr. K. was more firm than Mrs. K., often telling Patricia to "shape up," while Mrs. K. tended to indulge Patricia. Mrs. K. was more often at home and more often involved with Patricia. It seemed that both Patricia and Mrs. K. occasionally expressed mild disagreement with Mr. K. but they both feared doing so and instead ended up going along with his decisions. This was not a problem for any of them but it seemed worth noting at the time as a systemic situation which could help to account for, or be used to help alleviate, the presenting problem.

Suspecting that Patricia's interest in the religious aspects of the religious camp might represent a betrayal of the family's belief system, the author inquired about the parents' religion, about the degree to which Patricia had embraced the beliefs espoused by the camp's religious order, and about how the parents had felt about it. It seemed that Patricia had not embraced but had shown some heightened interest in this religious order due to her increased association with a particular friend who was a member of the order. Her father and mother had disapproved of this interest but mother had persuaded father to go along with allowing Patricia to go to the camp because she had hoped that Patricia would have fun and that it would do no harm.

The author also questioned Patricia about her symptoms, her interests, and her history. She gave the physical and psychological appearance of being slightly youngish for the age of 12, resembling a 10 or 11 year old. Her demeanor was soft and cooperative rather than defiant. She seemed to have a history of being impressionable and there were indications that she had a rich and active fantasy life. She tried hard to be obedient at home but often "forgot" or was "lazy." Peer relationships appeared appropriate for her developmental stage. She was clearly tormented by her symptom of hallucinations and wished to be rid of them.

During this conversation with Patricia, the author inquired about the specific content of the hallucinations. He found out that the hallucinations consisted only of auditory rather than other sorts of perceptual distortions, that they involved the voice of Sledge and no one else, and that the voice always sounded hostile, utilizing profanities which Patricia would not dare to use aloud. The content sometimes consisted of Sledge warning her that family members would die if she did not come with him. A second type of content consisted of Sledge telling Patricia that she did not have to listen to her father or to teachers, during those moments in which she was being instructed, lectured, or reprimanded. A third type of content consisted of Sledge telling Patricia to kill herself because she was "no good." Further questioning about this suicidal content revealed that Patricia felt she should kill herself both because she was evil and also because she was worthless for not being capable of controlling her symptoms.

By this point, the author had formulated several working hypotheses which provided direction for a series of therapeutic probes and interventions. He believed that the emergence in Patricia of normal adolescent urges to disobey and to individuate may have met with fear of defying her father and losing her family. This may have resulted in an exaggerated version of a typical adolescent conflict between the wish to separate from the family and a need to remain a child.

This conflict was actualized by Patricia's stay at the religious camp, which represented a move toward individuation and a betrayal of the family, a move which generated an intolerable degree of anxiety in Patricia. She was also a homesick and impressionable child who had been significantly traumatized by her camp experience. This was an experience which had put "ideas in her head," a common complaint made by many parents whose children enter alternate spheres of influence. The problem of hallucinations might also have been metaphoric for problematic interactions between the parents or for problems within the parents, such as headaches and health problems or inhibited wishes to defy authority. These ideas were far from confirmed at this point, but they were compatible with one another and rendered the author confident enough to proceed with interventions which he felt could be effective.

In terms of specific therapeutic goals, it was clear at this point that the symptom of hallucinations had too much power in the family and had to be rendered impotent or brought under control in some way. The symptom created an incongruous hierarchy in that the parents, physicians, nurses, and psychiatrist, who played the roles of helping and protecting Patricia, were rendered helpless in trying to control the problems. Second, the parental interaction around the management of the children and around the symptom was quite possibly relevant, but it was unknown in exactly what ways. Therefore, it was necessary to avoid tampering with this interaction until its relevance was more clear and necessary instead to preserve it in a temporary solution to the problem.

Prescribing the symptom. The first thing the author did was to request that Patricia experience the symptom of hallucination. He did this by first asking whether Sledge was at this moment speaking to her. Patricia responded that Sledge was not there at the moment. When asked if he was there but not speaking, she responded that she was not sure. The author asked her to close her eyes and to open them only when she knew Sledge was present because the author wanted Sledge to speak to Patricia. She closed her eyes and opened them a few moments later. When asked if she could hear him, she responded that he was listening but not speaking and that she did not wish him to speak because this was why she was in the hospital, where she did not want to be, wanting to be home instead.

The author explained that if he could help her to control when the voice spoke to her, then getting rid of the voice would also be under more control. She responded by saying that Sledge refused to speak because he knew what the author was trying to do. She looked down at this point, so the author asked her to look at him and to listen, and then waited a moment while Patricia directed her gaze and her attention on the author's face. He then clarified that Sledge knew that the author was trying to trick Sledge, and Patricia nodded to confirm this. The author pointed out that this was true and that he could indeed trick Sledge and get him to start talking because Sledge did not like the author or other grown-ups and always told Patricia not to listen to them, and that she could let the author know when she started to hear his voice because the author wanted to know what he was saying.

Patricia interrupted to say that Sledge was talking but that he did not want her to share what he was saying with the author. The author said that it was good that Sledge was telling her not to listen to the author because this was just what the author had said would happen. He pointed out that it was what Sledge usually did, and that Patricia could listen to Sledge all she liked; but that she would not be able to help listening to the author either, and neither could Sledge help it. Also, he emphasized that Sledge did not like it that the author had helped her to get him to speak against his will because it showed that Sledge was not so strong and powerful and that everyone present in the room was stronger.

She was then asked what Sledge had just been saying to her. She reported that he was continuing to tell her not to listen and was using profanity. The author said that this was good, and that she should now let herself hear him as clearly and as vividly as she ever did and to tell the author when she could hear him as clearly as the author's own voice. She was told to close her eyes if this would help. She did close her eyes and after a moment's silence she opened them and reported that she could hear Sledge vividly. The author further questioned her to confirm that it was as clear as a real voice.

He then told her that he was probably exhausting her with all of this and that she could now rest for a moment. He said he wanted to do something even more important in a moment and that she should let him know when Sledge had stopped talking. After a few moments she reported that Sledge had stopped talking. Inquiries to make certain of this revealed that he was still listening. The author told her to just rest a moment and gather her strength for the next stage.

The parent requests that the child have the problem. The author then turned to Mr. K. and asked whether he could see that some control over this voice was being achieved. Mr. K. looked pleased and agreed that he could see this happening. The author asked then if Mr. K. could now make the voice speak to Patricia and thereby control the voice, by means of pretending to get angry with Patricia.

The author pointed out that Mr. K. must know how to do this because he must have become angry with her from time to time. Mr. K. and Patricia both laughed, saying there certainly were times when this happened. Mr. K. was then asked if he could pretend to get angry now and to lecture or yell at Patricia, perhaps about school. He was told to only pretend, but to sound "real mean" so that he could be convincing enough to get that voice to start telling Patricia not to listen to her father and to call her father names.

Patricia interrupted to say that this would not work because Sledge was listening and knew what was being planned. The author said to her that Sledge could listen all he liked but that he could indeed be made to talk, and in fact could not help doing so. She was reminded that the author had helped her to control the voice and suggested to her that her father could now learn how to help her do this. She was told to let everyone know when her father had been effective in getting Sledge to talk to her.

Mr. K. was then asked to give her a good talking-to. He was coached to sound "mean" and convincing enough that Sledge would have no choice but to begin talking. Once Sledge began to speak to Patricia, the author ended this stage of the intervention by congratulating Mr. K. on being able to control Sledge. He told Mr. K. that he would be able to do this again if Patricia ever again complained of hearing voices; instead of being ambushed as helpless victims of this symptom, they could ambush the symptom by bringing the symptom on at times of their own choosing, thus proving their control over it. When Patricia was then asked who she now believed was more powerful, she indicated that her father was stronger than Sledge.

Use of ritual to externalize the hallucination. The author then initiated the next stage of the intervention by suggesting to Patricia that she allow herself to hear voices as clearly and as vividly as she wished while something very important was being accomplished. He then reached into his pocket and pulled out three tiny dolls, one of them a little girl and two of them adult male dolls. He then held them up and showed them to her. The incongruous and unexpected sight of these dolls riveted her attention. He told her that one of the male dolls could be Sledge. He asked her which looked most like Sledge and could really become him in her imagination. With great interest, she immediately reached out for the dolls, which were handed to her. After examining them she indicated which one was Sledge and was told to hold that doll in one hand and to give back the other.

The author then held up the doll of a little girl and told her that this could be Patricia, but only a certain part of Patricia: the bad part and worthless part that she wished to kill whenever she wished to kill herself. She was asked whether she understood that this represented, and could become, those bad parts that she wished to kill, but only the bad and worthless parts, and not the rest of herself. She indicated that she understood. She was handed this doll and told to hold it in her other hand.

Then she was reminded that she could tell when Sledge was present and when he was not, and that she could allow herself to hear the voice of Sledge as vividly as she liked or to know that he was listening, but that when she was really ready to get rid of him she could close her eyes and begin to squeeze the Sledge doll. As she squeezed tighter and tighter, it was suggested that Sledge would leave her and travel through her arm and into the doll. She then closed her eyes and began squeezing the doll while the author repeated the suggestion. He emphasized that she could stop squeezing when the voice was completely emptied out of her and present only in the doll. When she stopped squeezing and opened her eyes, she was asked to notice that she was sure that Sledge was no longer present, not even listening. She indicated she was sure, and that Sledge was in the doll.

She was then told to close her eyes and take all the time she needed to notice the parts of herself that she wished to kill, the parts that were bad and worthless. Then it was suggested that she begin squeezing the little girl doll, because as she squeezed, these parts could leave her and travel into the doll and be completely there and completely gone from herself until she no longer needed to wish to kill herself. She closed her eyes and began to squeeze and the author repeated these suggestions until she opened her eyes.

The author then asked if she could notice that she was sure where the bad and worthless parts of herself were and where Sledge was. She responded by indicating she was sure they were in the dolls and not within her any longer. The author asked her to close her eyes once again and to squeeze, just to be sure that any last parts of them were drained out and stop when she was positive. She closed her eyes and squeezed for a few seconds and then said she was done.

Problem substitution. Now the author told her that since Sledge and certain parts of her were no longer within her, that she would have to use the dolls to act out what she had been hearing before and that she would have to say aloud what she had only thought to herself before. An example was given of having the Sledge doll say to the little girl doll that she was bad and that she couldn't get rid of her problems, and that because of these things she should kill herself; and having the little girl doll answer something back. She responded by beginning to manipulate the dolls without speaking aloud, which suggested that she was only thinking through the dialogue; therefore, she was stopped and coached to speak it aloud until she grasped the idea and was able to implement it on her own. Her mother was advised to watch her and, when she did not play as instructed, to coach her to play with the dolls properly. Her father was asked to also encourage her doll play, but that when she actually played with the dolls he was to pretend to be annoyed that she was not acting her age.

The author then suggested to her that she could begin to notice that she was developing an urge to play like this with the dolls, an irresistible urge which she wouldn't be able to control, and that she could find herself wanting to play like this with the dolls more and more often. He said that he doubted she would enjoy this problem very much because it would make her appear younger than her age, very much like a baby or a little girl. He also said that her parents would probably find the doll play annoying because it would happen more and more often and would come to have the appearance of being a problem. Although she would act babyish while playing with the dolls, it was implied that she would probably act her age when not involved with the doll play. The author said that he wondered how long it would take before she realized she wanted to play with the dolls more and more often. He also said that he wondered how long it would take before everyone saw that she was playing with the dolls more and more often, because at that point everyone would know for sure that the voices were gone and that her problem was now one of wanting to play with dolls like a baby. At that point, she was told, she would be ready to leave the hospital.

Reframing the reality of hallucinations. The author switched topics, to prevent the previous hour's content from being analyzed too carefully and to preserve the potency of the therapeutic suggestions. The new topic was intended to contain suggestions which would help to make this intervention appear to be less ''magical'' in the future upon retrospection and to provide Patricia with a guide and perspective for how to view and use her imaginative capacity. The author talked about how powerful Patricia's imagination was, how it could amuse her with vivid and pleasant daydreams and how it could also torment her with nightmarish fantasies. He asked her to close her eyes and imagine hearing the song ''Jingle Bells'' and to tell him when she could actually hear the voice of someone singing it.

She closed her eyes and a few moments later reported that she could hear her father singing. The author complimented her. He said that everyone could hear voices when they dreamed and some people could hear their thoughts as voices when very fatigued after a hard day or when using drugs, but only a few had imaginations so strong that they could do this as easily as she could while wide awake. He pointed out that an imagination so strong and vivid could make a voice out of any thought one might have and that this could make it difficult to avoid confusing what was real with what was imaginary. He repeated that an imagination so strong could be a great source of torment but also could become a great source of comfort if she learned how to use it efficiently. He pointed out that she had begun to learn to do this in the past hour.

Finalizing the intervention. Patricia again asked when she would be permitted to leave. The author said he was unsure because that was up to her and how soon the irresistible urge developed to play with dolls like a baby. She argued that she already had the urge and was therefore ready to leave and that she really wanted to go home. The author replied that he knew she wanted to go home very badly but that right now everyone should take a short break before talking any more about things because Patricia had been through an exhausting experience in the past hour or so. In the brief everyday conversation that followed in the next minute, Patricia did say how tired she was but also indicated that her headache was gone.

The author and the psychiatrist then left the room and conferred with the staff pediatrician who would be responsible for discharging Patricia. It was decided that she would be discharged only when she had convincingly demonstrated to her parents and to hospital staff that she had developed a habit of playing with the dolls. This criterion would ensure that the intervention had taken hold prior to discharge; if it did not take hold, she would still be safe in the hospital until the intervention could be modified. It was also decided that she would be taken off all medications; in addition to the Mellaril, she had been taking medication for her headaches.

The author and the psychiatrist then returned to Patricia's hospital room. Mrs. K. immediately asked the author whether it was normal for a teenager to play with dolls; the reason she asked was that she permitted it with Patricia's older sisters, but her husband disapproved and expected those daughters to act their age. This information helped to confirm that the parents tended to interact in a particular way around issues involving the children; it also confirmed the importance of preserving that interaction in the temporary solution until the interaction was better understood.

The author emphasized that this problem of playing with dolls was only a temporary solution but could continue at least until the next meeting. It was suggested again that Mrs. K. should remind Patricia to play with the dolls if that were necessary and to encourage and indulge the play. At the same time, Mr. K. was to pretend to act tough and to look annoyed with Patricia, telling her to "shape up and act your age." The parents could even pretend to argue about this issue of whether Patricia should be allowed to play with dolls at her age. If the voices should recur, Mr. K. was asked to prove that he was more powerful than the voices by means of the tactic he had learned earlier, but this back-up measure would be unnecessary if the voices did not recur.

When Patricia again asked when she could go home, the criterion for discharge was made clear to her again. She responded with desperate wailing, begging to be allowed to go home and not have to stay another night. She pleaded that she already had an urge to play with the dolls and wanted to play with them all the time; she also promised to play with them all the time when she got home if she could be discharged now. It was difficult for the author and the psychiatrist to remain firm in the onslaught of that heartwrenching performance, but they calmly, firmly, and repeatedly explained that some time was necessary for everyone to be able to observe her playing with dolls and to become convinced that she had developed a new problem; he again said he wondered how soon this would be.

The author then asked to see the parents in another room for a few minutes. His purpose for this meeting was to be sure that they were comfortable with what had transpired and with the plan for the near future. When asked about this, they responded that they were comfortable with whatever "got results" and the intervention thus far seemed to be accomplishing this. Mrs. K. also expressed appreciation for eliminating her own headache, which had suddenly vanished after she had suffered with it for some time. The author had not known she had headaches, since he had earlier formulated the mistaken hypothesis that it was the father who had the headaches.

Mrs. K. also asked whether it would be useful to use hypnotism for Patricia's problem. The author responded that hypnotic methods had just been used. Mrs. K. said that she had thought so, and she appeared to be satisfied with this information. She also revealed the interesting information that Patricia often seemed to be in trances and that she had to be shaken, or distracted, out of them. She also sometimes had trance-like expressions on her face when she worked herself into believing that terrible things she worried would happen had really happened.

Mr. and Mrs. K. were asked if they had any questions about the plan because it was important for them to understand it well enough to implement it properly. They were also asked if they had the strength to carry out the plan, no matter how heartwrenching Patricia's pleading became, and they said that they did. As the author and the psychiatrist left, Patricia's desperate wailing could be heard down the halls.

Subsequent sessions. Patricia stayed in the hospital that night and by the next day had played with the dolls enough for the pediatrician to discharge her. She and her parents met with the author and the psychiatrist a few days later in the psychiatrist's office. The plan for this second meeting was to monitor progress and provide further interventions which might be indicated by the situation. The family reported that all was going well and that the voice of Sledge had not returned. Patricia was playing with her dolls and was carrying them on her person wrapped in a handkerchief. She appeared child-like when playing with the dolls but was otherwise engaging in age-appropriate activities. She was asked to continue the doll play every day until the next meeting. It was emphasized that the family should "not get too happy" about the changes because only temporary measures had been taken to resolve the problems thus far. There were still school problems to address and there was a need to influence any factors that may have contributed to and maintained the problem of hearing voices.

The author then explained to the family that part of the problem was a normal adolescent conflict between a wish to remain a child and the need to separate and individuate. Due to Patricia's love and respect for her parents, she was fearful of admitting, even to herself, some of the usual kinds of wishes and urges experienced by adolescents which might be construed as defiance. The author went on to explain that it could be useful for Patricia to learn that she could attempt to defy her father without fearing that she would lose him. He pointed out that her father could tolerate this and still be able to keep her in line. She would have to sacrifice a bit by suffering her father's punishments and anger in order to learn this important lesson.

The author and the psychiatrist then met with Patricia alone, followed by a short meeting with the parents. Areas of mild disobedience were explored and Patricia was coached to behave disobediently in mild circumscribed ways. She was very fearful and reluctant to do so but agreed to try. The parents were coached to allow her some expression of rebellion in these circumscribed areas but to hold her accountable for her actions, and to do so in a way that allowed her to learn that a step towards defiance was not the end of the world. They were all told that they should get used to this because this was what much of adolescence was about and that this topic could be discussed further at subsequent meetings.

The next meeting was held two weeks later. Patricia had disobeyed in some mild ways and her parents had attempted to catch her at her acts of disobedience. The parents felt that they were still in charge of Patricia's behavior and she was learning that urges towards defiance and individuation were not catastrophic. Patricia had also continued to engage in age-appropriate activities, such as going to dances and having friends to the house. She had not experienced any further hallucinations nor any suicidal ideation. She had continued to play with the dolls but felt weary of this exercise and wished to stop, although she made it clear that she would continue if it was required.

The author informed the family that the doll play was no longer necessary because the voices had stopped torturing Patricia, but that some measure should be taken to deal with voices if they should recur. He told the family that they could cover the dolls with a handkerchief and then put them in an old box and to cover the box; this should then be hidden away in a drawer or cupboard for safekeeping. They were also to store with it a piece of paper containing a monologue written by the author. If the voices recurred, Mr. K. could get the dolls, hand them to Patricia, and then read the monologue to her.

The monologue would consist of detailed suggestions for Patricia to close her eyes and to allow the voices to leave her and enter the dolls, in words almost identical to those used by the author in the hospital. The author then wrote out the monologue and gave it to Mr. K. The family members understood and felt comfortable with this task. The author informed them that he was no longer necessary, since the voices were gone. He said that the psychiatrist would continue meeting with them to work on school problems and on other family problems concerning Patricia.

Following this third meeting with the family, the author did not meet with the family again, stepping out of the situation as soon as the purpose for which his help was requested had been accomplished. He did provide consultation to the psychiatrist from time to time and stayed in touch with the case. At a four month follow-up call, the hallucinations and suicidal ideation had not recurred. The therapy was focused on Patricia's difficulty in concentrating in school, on educational planning, and on family management of her behavior. At a nine month follow-up, the hallucinations and suicidal ideation had still not recurred and the therapy was now focussed on mild acting out by Patricia and on problematic interaction in the family.

Discussion

The rationales for the interventions used in this case are discussed below. However, in order to adequately discuss these rationales, it could be helpful to readers unfamiliar with Madanes (1981) to review her strategic family therapy approach to problems involving children. The approach will be described here in enough detail so that it will be evident that its theoretical rationale involving hierarchical incongruity bears an equivalence to the hypnotic relationship. This equivalence illustrates the interface that is established between the therapist and the problem, an interface that is more apparent in the case example of this chapter than in many other cases.

Madanes' approach. Madanes identified six strategies for resolving problems with young children. The strategies are based on the hypothesis that a symptom has a protective function in a family, distracting the parents from their own problems and bringing out the parental best in them. Whether or not this hypothesis is supported by fact, it is a refreshing alternative to some of the more common working hypotheses in family therapy approaches. The hypothesis implies that the symptom has a benevolent function; it also leads to several innovative and playful interventions.

This hypothesis is not a simple one; it can be viewed as a multi-faceted proposition or as a broad theoretical orientation. It consists, first, of the proposition that a child's symptom is a metaphor or an analogy for a problem that one of the parents have or for a problematic interaction between the parents. This metaphoric component helps to account for the specificity of symptoms, that is, why a symptom might consist of headaches rather than a phobia or some other specific content. For example, a child's headaches might be metaphoric for the father's "headaches on the job." The symptom's function is to distract the parent from his own problem and to get the parent to rise to the occasion of attempting to help the child. Thus, rather than the parent being overwhelmed by his own problems, the best is brought out of him as a parent in the attempt to protect and help the child. These protective and helping behaviors define him as hierarchically superior to the overwhelmed, symptomatic child.

This is an unfortunate solution because it results in a hierarchical incongruity: although the parent is in a superior position by virtue of playing the role of helping the symptomatic child, he is nevertheless powerless in his attempts to remove the child's symptoms, which in this respect are more powerful than the parent. Thus, in this respect, the child is more powerful than the parent but simultaneously he is less powerful because he is helpless in regard to his symptom; the parent is also simultaneously powerful yet helpless. Finally, a further incongruity exists on another level, which may be evident from what had already been said above: the power to help or protect the parent, by having a symptom, serves to put the child in a superior, protective position to the parent, which is incongruous with the usual hierarchical relationship in which the parent helps and protects the child.

These incongruities are important to consider because according to this theoretical view, a person who is simultaneously defined as powerful and helpless, by his relationships and interactions with others, will behave in symptomatic ways which represent the incongruous hierarchy in which he is involved. He will develop a symptom too powerful for others to control and in regard to which he feels helpless, believing he has no voluntary control over it. According to this view, when one person is powerful but helpless, others with whom he interacts must interact accordingly in a way that is also powerful but helpless.

The system of interaction around a problem is also viewed as analogical or metaphorical for another or a previous system of interaction in the family. Thus, a father's helpful, reassuring behavior in regard to a child's headaches may be analogical for the mother's previous habit of reassuring the father in regard to his job difficulties; or the parent's disagreement concerning the management of a child's tantrums might be analogical for a conflict between them which neither feel it is safe to explicitly discuss anymore. If attention were to remain on the original interactions, the disrupted power balance between the parents would become painfully evident and might threaten the relationship; for example, father's insecurity on the job might put him in a one-down position in regard to his wife, disrupting a delicate power balance in a way which neither of them understands or knows how to address. A problem in a child can then serve to distract the parents from their problem, empower the father, restore a power balance, and preserve, analogically, other interactions in the family.

From these ideas, a number of interesting strategies were developed which were aimed at resolving hierarchical incongruities and removing the need for, or function of, the symptom. Several are relevant to the case of Patricia K. because the author adapted these to the circumstances of the case. For example, in one strategy, which best illustrates Madanes' "pretend" approaches, the parents pretend to have a problem similar to the child's and the child pretends to help the parent with it.

In this strategy, the parent is now playing a helpless role, but the "pretended" helplessness implies the opposite of helplessness, thus restoring a single hierarchy. The child no longer needs to have a symptom to help the parent. What each of them pretends serves this purpose and is enough to become a focus of concern. The symptom is stripped of its power because it no longer has a function. Previously it denoted, or was metaphorical for, a problem in a parent and served to help the parent. Now the pretended behavior has no real influence on the original problem in the parents. While pretending to have a symptom denotes or is metaphorical for the symptom, it does not denote, or is not metaphorical for the problem in the parents which the symptom denoted.

The same effects are intended in another strategy in which the parent requests that the child pretend to have the problem. Because it is pretend, the pretended problem is analogical for the problem but no longer analogical for the original problem in the parents. In the same way as was described in the previous strategy, a single hierarchy is restored in which the parent is in charge of the child. Madanes also includes a standard paradoxical strategy in which the parent requests that the child actually have the problem.

Another strategy is relevant here and was identified by Madanes as "changing the metaphorical action." A child's symptom is again viewed as metaphorical for another problem and considered to be an unfortunate and painful solution for that problem. The intent of the intervention is to replace the symptom with another ritualistic behavior which is not as painful as the symptom itself but which will fulfill some of the same purposes.

For example, Erickson replaced a boy's compulsion to pick at a sore with a compulsion to write accurately (Haley, 1973); other examples include replacing a child's compulsion to stick pins in his stomach with a compulsion to stick pins in a doll (Madanes, 1981) and replacing a child's wild horseplay with competent and skillful wrestling (Hoorwitz, 1985). If necessary, important aspects of the interaction around the symptom can be preserved by this substitution of one behavior for another. If the parent is put in charge of seeing to it that the child perform the therapeutic task, rather than trying unsuccessfully to remove the symptom, a single hierarchy can be restored.

Working hypotheses for the intervention. Although other interesting and useful strategies were identified by Madanes, the four reviewed here are the ones most relevant to the case of Patricia. There was an integrated use of these rather than a pure application of any of them. These sorts of intervention were considered appropriate for use due to the nature of the author's working hypotheses about the problem.

It seemed clear that Mr. and Mrs. K., accustomed to feeling in charge of their children, felt helpless in their attempts to overcome the problem of Patricia's hallucinations. Her hallucinations, while causing her great torment, had a great deal of power to elicit helpful but futile action from everyone concerned. Escalation of symptomatic behavior by Patricia was met by escalations of helpful behavior by parents, physicians, teachers, and therapists; this symmetrical escalation suggested the possibility that attempts to solve the problem were serving to maintain it. This is a frequent and useful working hypothesis of the MRI approach to strategic therapy (Fisch et al., 1982). This seemed to be intuitively evident upon observing the panic and helplessness that seemed to motivate the helping behavior of the helpers. It was clear that the usual helping behavior had to be blocked and that the interpersonal meaning or communicative function of the symptom had to be altered.

It was unclear whether the symptom was metaphoric for a problem between the parents or for a problem that one of them had, but this was considered possible. For example, it was hypothesized that headaches or health problems might exist in one of the parents. It was also considered possible that the hallucinations, the content of which reflected conflicts concerning defiance and separation, were metaphoric for wishes in one or the other parent to defy or separate from the other. The interaction between the parents concerning the problem also seemed relevant because it was analogical for a frequent form of interaction in this family. Mr. K. was more firm than Mrs. K., usually having the last word on important decisions. Mrs. K. was more indulgent and the children tended to get their way with her. She also played the role of extracting from Mr. K. his reluctant permission for the children to engage in activities of which he did not approve.

It was not necessary to confirm or disconfirm the more uncertain of the hypotheses noted above. The interventions which were used were intended to capitalize on them if they were valid but did not depend on them if they were invalid. The interventions depended more on the validity of three other hypotheses: that Patricia possessed imaginative capacities which produced vivid images; that she had been traumatized by the camp experience as hypothesized by her parents; and that she was struggling with developmental conflicts concerning defiance and separation.

The hypothesis about a developmental crisis was suggested by Mr. K.'s reluctance to allow Patricia to go to a camp whose religious ideas were discrepant with the family's, by Patricia's appearance of exaggerated child-like obedience, by her anxious fascination with the ideas presented at the religious camp, and by the content of her hallucinations. The content of one of the hallucinations consisted of a confused and illogical threat: "Come with me or your family dies." This content is confused in the sense that it is discrepant with reality. It can be translated to "If you separate from your family, they will live," which is discrepant from her fear while at camp that harm could come to them if she was away from them. It can also be translated to, "If you stay at home, your family will die," which is discrepant with the above noted fear and with the security she experienced at home.

At least two incongruous messages are combined in a way which put

Patricia in a bind: stay and they die, or leave and they die. It was probably a confused message because it reflected a conflict about separation; that is, a wish and fear to leave home, combined with a wish and a reluctance to remain a child at home. She was able to avoid addressing this very difficult, but typical conflict of adolescence by developing a symptom which demanded she leave home but which resulted in a developmental regression that permitted her to stay at home where she was treated like a "sick" or younger child.

The content of another of the hallucinations provides some support for the notion that typical adolescent struggles were pertinent. The voice telling her she did not have to listen to adult authority resembles the classic angel-devil dialogues in which one ear hears the voice of virtue saying that it is better not to taste the forbidden fruit and the other ear hears the voice of temptation. In this hallucination, Patricia seemed to be hearing the voice of normal adolescent feelings and urges which she feared to acknowledge in herself.

Combining these various hypotheses, the author believed Patricia to have been an impressionable child with a vivid imagination, sheltered and loyal to her family, and experiencing normal urges to individuate. Her camp experience represented to her a betrayal of her family as a first step at separation, and this prospect of separation was too anxiety provoking for her to bear. The camp experience was also traumatic due to her being impressionable and possibly due to the ideas to which she was exposed. The metaphor of people "putting ideas in your head" which is feared by the parents of many adolescents was literally realized here. The author considered Patricia's problem to be metaphorical for the complicated and general process of an adolescent growing up in a family, leaving home, and being exposed to and not equipped for the insults of this world. It might have been metaphoric for much else as well, as has been noted previously, but the author was not as certain of this.

The interventions. The most prominent portion of the author's intervention consisted of the exorcism of voices using dolls and the suggestion for regressive doll play. While these two portions may have been the most important, the author's direct involvement in the therapy can be viewed as a stage-wise intervention, consisting of about seven stages. The first stage consisted of joining with the family, achieving rapport, and assessment.

The second stage consisted of a paradoxical prescription of the hallucinations in order to gain control over them. It was similar, though not identical, to Madanes' strategy of having the parent request that the child have the symptom. Unlike previous attempts to address Patricia's problem, consisting of behaviors by helping persons which did not help and which may have instead served to maintain the problem, this approach side-stepped Patricia's interactional style of engaging helpers in fruitless struggles. Instead, it confronted the problem head-on by requesting that it make an appearance. This altered the functions that it usually had in other interactional contexts; aside from altering its transactional meaning, the author was able to establish control over it, which was important for subsequent stages. This strategy served as an experimental probe which assessed whether the author was on the right track and could continue to proceed in the direction he did. If this step had failed or proceeded differently, subsequent interventions would probably have been different.

In the third stage of intervention, the control over the hallucinations which the author had achieved was shared with, or transferred to, Mr. K. The way in which this was accomplished was similar, again, to the Madanes strategy of the parent requesting that the child have the problem. Yet, it was also similar to Madanes' "pretend" strategies in that Mr. K. was asked to pretend to be stern with Patricia in order to elicit the problem. The playfulness engendered by pretending probably helped to buffer the pain attendant on experiencing unwanted hallucinations. It resulted in a re-enactment of what usually occurred in the family and at school, but it now occurred in a different interactional context that would alter the transactional meaning of the problem. Instead of Mr. K. being powerless when the symptom occurred, he was now more powerful than the symptom because he could control it by intentionally eliciting it. This realigned the hierarchical incongruity, restoring the relationship to a single hierarchy. It was hoped that this demonstration of Mr. K.'s power would be dramatic enough to Patricia so that further demonstrations at home would be unnecessary.

The author did not trust that these two interventions described above would eliminate the symptom. He worried that they did not encompass enough of the symptom's forms of appearance to prevent a re-emergence and a restoration of the symptom's power. Therefore he decided to use hypnotic methods to facilitate a redefinition of ego boundaries and of reality. He did this by suggesting that Patricia could exorcise the hallucinations and by suggesting that she could develop a problem of regressed behavior. These interventions constituted the fourth and fifth stages. By this time the author trusted Patricia's imaginative capacity enough to believe that these goals could be accomplished without having to use formal procedures of trance induction or trance deepening.

The introduction of the dolls was incongruous enough to the situation that it riveted Patricia's attention. It was also incongruous and exotic enough to emphasize a strong but implicit message which was being conveyed by the therapist's behavior that whatever procedures were about to be used would be effective in eliminating her problem. As has been noted in previous chapters, this is a hypnotic message conveyed in the use of any ritual. The message is that if this ritual is performed, a curative response will occur. The implication is that the person should give up conscious efforts to cure the problem because by engaging in the ritual, the curative response will occur on its own without conscious efforts to produce it.

The use of dolls probably appealed to the child in her, especially to those cognitive capacities that enabled her to regress to a preoperational stage of logic where magical thinking creates a magical reality (O'Connor, 1984). This stage is one where pretend and play can seem real, where hallucination and delusion are normal, where syncretic logic dominates, and where thought of an action can become confused with having actually performed the action. The author also thought it possible that Patricia had been exposed to exorcism rituals on television and that she would believe as much in an exotic ritual of this kind as she did in the reality of her hallucinations. It also occurred to the author that this was the kind of intervention Mrs. K. may have had in mind in her previous requests for hypnotism. The specific suggestions which the author made were similar to hypnotic suggestions which might be used to achieve any hypnotic effects. For example, the suggestion ". . . as you squeeze harder and harder, the voice will leave you and go into the doll. . . " is equivalent in form to ". . . as you stare at the dot on the wall, your eyelids will feel heavier and heavier."

The author went slowly through this stage, in several steps, first exorcising Sledge, then a part of Patricia, then taking precautions to be certain the exorcism was complete. This step-by-step pace was necessary to ratify the effects of each step, both for the author and for Patricia, helping both of them to understand that each step had been successful and increasing belief in the probability of success for subsequent steps. The author thought it would be safest to also exorcize or externalize that part of Patricia which she wished to kill and which she thought was "bad"; this was intended as a temporary measure, not as a final solution. As a temporary measure, it would help reduce the probability of suicidal thoughts, by containing them in the doll, a vehicle which Patricia believed could indeed contain them. Free now of both hallucinations and the "bad" girl in her, she could now be the "good little girl" she wished to be, which would enable her to get out of the hospital, go home, and feel symptom free.

However, the author believed that this goal was itself regressive and symptomatic, constituting one side of an adolescent conflict between dependence and independence in regard to the family. Therefore, as part of this family's reality, this side of the conflict could be exaggerated and used to transform the problem from that of hallucinations and suicidal ideation to one of regression in development. This was equivalent to Madanes' strategy of "altering the metaphorical action," and can be identified as the fifth stage in the intervention. The alteration is from a painful problem which the family is helpless to control to a more manageable and less painful problem. In this case, it was important that the alteration continue to constitute a problem, that is, appear odd, abnormal, and be inconvenient to those involved, in order to provide a reminder for the need for continued therapy and to preserve the imperfectly understood interaction around the problem (that is, father telling Patricia to shape up and mother being more indulgent).

In order to render the doll play unnecessary, an attempt was made in the sixth stage of the intervention to help Patricia to believe that defiant wishes were acceptable and could be acknowledged, as long as her defiant behavior remained within certain limits. The voices and the suicidal ideation did not recur and the family seemed to be getting on with its life, hopefully evolving patterns of interaction which maintained symptom-free behavior. Therefore, the author's intervention no longer appeared necessary.

In the intervention's final stage, the dolls were buried and put to rest in a ritualistic manner that put closure on the problem of hallucinations and suicide. Yet, this burial preserved the power of these dolls and of previous hypnotic suggestions should they ever be required again. The way this was done served to empower the parents to deal with the problem effectively on a temporary basis, if it should recur, until they could arrange for therapeutic assistance. Factors which were still unclear or which might require further intervention were left for the psychiatrist to explore, such as teaching Patricia to use the power of her imagination more constructively, adolescent conflicts, problematic interaction in the family, school problems, and so on.

Therapeutic interface with the problem. To some extent, the effectiveness of the interventions here has been attributed to the restoration of a single hierarchy in the family; also, the problem was viewed as an unfortunate means by which a hierarchical incongruity was maintained. One reason for devoting so much discussion to a set of strategic interventions which depend on notions of hierarchical incongruity and incongruous messages is that the hypnotic relationship can be understood in the same terms. In a case like this there is a clear interface between the system which consists of the hypnotic relationship and the system in which the symptomatic behavior is embedded, an interface which occurs in most other cases as well but much less clearly.

It was said earlier that when a person is involved in a hierarchical incongruity, or receives incongruous or contradictory messages, then that person may behave in symptomatic ways which reflect the incongruity. The problem will be one which is too powerful for others to control, despite their helpful efforts to do so, and also one over which the person has no voluntary control. When the person then behaves in ways which are powerful but helpless in interactions with others, others tend to behave in a similarly incongruous fashion. The problem, which is unfortunate and painful, is maintained or produced by messages which are contradictory or incongruous in the same way that a hypnotic response, which is usually desirable and nonpainful, is produced by contradictory or incongruous messages to change but not to change on purpose.

The hypnotist does not allow the subject to respond to only one of the two incongruous messages because a response to only one level would be either symmetrical or complementary and not hypnotic. A hypnotic response is one in which the person performs a response, such as hallucination, but indicates in some way that she is not doing so on purpose. The subject's orientation to the hypnotic response is the same as a client's orientation to a symptomatic response; it is happening but not on purpose. In this way, a hypnotic response, whether it be that of arm levitation, relaxation, eye closure, amnesia, anesthesia, hallucination, or age regression, is equivalent to the production of a symptomatic response, such as Patricia's symptom of hallucinations. Each is a response to incongruous messages and in turn conveys incongruous messages. The therapist can employ this knowledge concerning the hypnotic relationship to form an interlocking relationship with a person's relationship to the symptomatic behavior. He does this by making incongruous demands which are congruous with the incongruous messages conveyed by the symptomatic behavior.

This congruity is the point of interface and it locks or checks the progress of the problem. The therapist is in the position of either 1) demanding that the client have the problem but not on purpose, or 2) demanding that the client get rid of the problem but not on purpose, or 3) demanding both of the above sequentially. This position contrasts with a usual, or normal, or nontherapeutic position of demanding that the client purposefully stop having the problem; it also contrasts with the position of resigning oneself to the existence of the problem and having no power to control it. The therapist's position is one which agrees with the client that the client cannot voluntarily control the symptom; in enforcing this agreement the therapist prevents a complementary relationship in which the production of the symptom would be defined as voluntary obedience and also prevents a symmetrical relationship in which a client's futile attempts to get rid of the symptom could be defined as resistance. The client is thereby helped to abandon a symmetrical struggle with the problem, a struggle which has only served to maintain the power of the problem and the client's powerlessness over it. The client's attention is directed away from this sort of struggle so that therapeutic suggestions for change can take hold.

Concluding Remarks

The congruous interface between a therapist's incongruous demands and the incongruous messages conveyed by symptomatic behavior is one that can be achieved in any therapy, therapies that are nonhypnotic as well as hyponotic. In this case, the interface readjusted the interactions and relationships in a family and in a larger system of helping agents, due to the way the symptomatic behavior was anchored in, and reflected, the incongruities in the interactions in those systems. The case also illustrates how aspects of this wider context can be employed to facilitate the interface. It makes clear that the integration of hypnotic methods in a family therapy approach is not simply the utilization of hypnosis in front of a family of observers, but rather the utilization and orchestration of family interaction to maximize the impact of hypnotic methods which facilitate change.

11

BRIEF CASE ILLUSTRATIONS

The extensive detail in the case illustrations of previous chapters was necessary to help clarify the nature of the integration of hypnotic methods in nonhypnotic contexts. In order to permit an appreciation of that integration, an emphasis was placed on describing those contexts in enough detail that the nonhypnotic aspects and the various forms of therapy used would be clear. The degree of detail also permitted a microscopic focus on the ways in which hypnotic principles can be applied. Since the purposes of this detailed illustration have been well enough met at this point, the present chapter will present a greater number of cases in a briefer form. The purpose is to better convey the diversity of contexts in which hypnotic methods can be applied. Many of the subtle aspects of therapist behavior have been omitted in some of these illustrations but they can be easily imagined on the basis of detailed illustrations in previous chapters.

The first few case presentations are rather brief. They are followed by some which are somewhat lengthier and more detailed, but which are not large enough to merit separate chapters. Since the chapter is so large and since some of the case presentations can be regarded as mini-chapters, the table of contents at the beginning of the book lists each case illustration in order to provide a convenient reference.

Case 1: An Obsessive Child

John J. was 10 years of age when he was brought to the author by his mother and stepfather. John was suffering from the effects of family disruption, the loss of his father, and the difficulties of adjusting in a new stepfamily. An approach was taken with the mother and stepfather which attempted to educate them about the effects of divorce and step-family readjustment. This education provided a foundation for their de-velopment of new solutions to practical problems and for a number of suggestions the author made which were intended to ameliorate various difficulties. The approach could be characterized as predominantly de-velopmental, structural, and educational.

After a few sessions, a number of significant changes had been made, but John seemed to be significantly distressed by obsessive ruminations which distracted him from school work and which diminished his pleasure in activities which he ordinarily enjoyed. He had been suffering from this problem for approximately six months. He ruminated about mistakes he may have made in the past and those he might make in the future. For example, if there was any chance that he might have left a backyard gate unlatched while leaving a friend's house, he might ruminate about this for hours, worrying that the gate might swing open in the wind and knock over an old lady who might be walking by, or that it might be an invitation to burglars, or that other imaginable catastrophes might result from this possible mistake. Various other mistakes from both the distant and recent past occupied his attention in this way.

He wished to get to the bottom of this problem by exploring his early childhood and his conflicts. The author agreed this might be useful and he did subsequently spend about a half dozen meetings with John ad-dressing his mishandling of anger, his perfectionism, and other issues which the author believed contributed to the problem. However, since the author did not know in advance how long this process of exploration would take, he told John that before beginning with this exploration he wished to teach John a method that would help him to control his habit of ruminating so much. That way John would not have to wait for an indefinite period while the exploration was underway before being able to concentrate in school and enjoying pleasurable activities once again. John seemed eager to learn a method that would accomplish this.

Since John now firmly believed that a method existed which would stop him from ruminating so much, it is possible that any method which was provided, even a placebo, would facilitate change. The method chosen was "thought-stopping", a cognitive-behavioral method which the author believed might have an impact on the problem aside from the effect of John's belief that change would occur.

While explaining the technical components of the method to John, the

author interspersed a number of suggestions conveying the message that
the method would be effective. Before leading John through the method,
the author first asked John to think of a powerful image of someone
commanding his ruminating to stop, for example, a stop sign, or a po-
liceman with his hand held up, or a train stop. He chose a soldier with
a big gun in one hand and the other hand held up with palm faced outward.
Second, John was asked to think of a pleasant scene which relaxed him,
and which helped him to feel happy and good about himself. He thought
of riding his bike on a bike-path along the river. Next, he was asked to
construct three statements about himself which identified positive characteristics about which he could feel proud, for example, "I'm pretty
good at sports compared to most kids my age."

Then he was taught the method, which consisted of a sequence of five
steps. The first step was to bring on the symptom. He asked why he
would ever want to do that. The author responded that he had to bring
on the symptom in order to practice the method and that the more he
practiced in a deliberate fashion, the more available the method would
be if the symptom ambushed him when he wasn't ready for it. He was
told that he could practice at the beginning with "mistakes" which were
very minor and which hardly troubled him at all, and then work up to
more distressing thoughts as he felt ready.

Since John was a military buff, the author told him about Sun Tsu,
an ancient military strategist, who advised in *The Art of War* that it was
wise to begin a battle when well rested and when the enemy was tired
from traveling. He was asked if it was wise to wait to use this thought-
stopping until he was ambushed by the symptom of rumination, an ambush that might occur when he was tired and not thinking about the
proper way to use thought-stopping; or whether it was wiser to practice
thought-stopping by ambushing the symptom when he felt prepared,
rested, and strong.

He seemed to like the military metaphor and replied that a good general
would ambush the symptom. He was then taught how to bring on the
symptom. The second step consisted of yelling "Stop," slapping his
knee, and picturing the soldier with the hand held up. John was told that
when he was in public he could whisper this subvocally so that only he
knew he was doing it and could put his hand in his trouser pocket and
press hard on his leg instead of slapping his knee.

In the third step, he was to clench his right hand into a fist and squeeze
for about 30 seconds as hard as he could until he could squeeze no harder.
This step was intended to distract him from the ruminating as well as

from the previous step which had also been intended to distract him from the ruminating. It was a second order distraction, or a distraction from a distraction. It also served to increase tension in order to provide a vivid counterpoint to, and a measure of, the relaxation that was to be suggested in the next step. The fourth step was to allow his hand to relax, little by little, for about 30 seconds. The fifth step was to imagine himself riding his bike along the river and saying three positive things about himself.

The author led John through a rehearsal of each step and then asked him to explain the sequence of the steps to the author. Then John was asked to apply the method himself in the session. Both times he practiced the method, first with the author's help and then on his own, it was clear from his behavior and physical appearance, that his imaginative involvement was equivalent to trance behavior.

He was asked to practice this method between one and five times a day. The author suggested that it might not work very well at first but that the more he practiced, by ambushing the symptom, the better he would become at it. The better he became at it, the more likely it was that it would be available as an effective weapon for when the symptom ambushed him. He was told to simply practice ambushing the symptom in the first week and not to feel like he had to do anything at all when the symptom ambushed him; instead he was simply to suffer as before and bide his time with the private knowledge that the development of a secret weapon was in progress.

By the next week he had practiced it sufficiently for it to be an effective weapon and, against the author's advice, he had even used it at times against ambushes. He reported that it was not completely successful in terminating his obsessive ruminations each and every time they ambushed him but that the frequency of their occurrence had dramatically decreased.

By detailed questioning, the author discovered that during ambushes, John was making the mistake of hesitating when he pictured the soldier saying "Stop." He was waiting for the ruminating to entirely cease before moving along to the hand clenching. The author suggested he move right along without hesitation in any future responses to ambush. It was also suggested to him that when he was ambushed, he should not immediately begin with the second step of yelling "Stop" and imagining the soldier. Instead, he was to begin with step one. Although he didn't have to actually bring on the symptom, since it had made its own appearance, he could at least make it a bit worse before he started getting rid of it. In this way, even though he was ambushed, he would be taking some control over the symptom from the outset and in some sense ambushing it in return.

By the following week, all ruminating had ceased and subsequent sessions focused on issues related to his obsessive cognitive style and his general development and adjustment. The symptom failed to make any reappearance through the course of therapy.

Case 2: Mental Retardation

As the consultant to a group home, the author was asked for help in devising a behavioral plan to help the residents to exit the building within a prescribed time after hearing a fire alarm. The plan was devised and implemented, with practice sessions occurring on a regular basis. The plan worked effectively with most residents, but some residents were developmentally disabled, with intellectual and adaptive ability in the range of profound mental retardation. They also suffered from sensory and physical handicaps. These residents were wholly unable to grasp the notion of what was required and engaged in oppositional and random behavior when prompted to exit from the building.

For example, after the alarm began to sound, a staff member would wait for a certain time period for the resident to get up from a sitting position on his bed. If the resident failed to rise, the staff would provide a verbal prompt and, after a certain time period, would then provide a physical prompt if the resident still had not moved. Sometimes the resident would rise. When the resident did not, he would be pulled to his feet. Then the resident would be led towards the bedroom door and down the hall towards the front door of the house. If the resident turned to the side or reversed direction, the staff would directly resist this and pull the resident in the desired direction. If the resident dropped to the floor, the staff would pull the resident to his or her feet.

The task had taken on the appearance of a tug of war, with residents displaying displeasure and staff members dreading the chore of causing unhappiness to the residents in this way. It had also become a boring and physically exhausting task for staff members. In addition, the residents were not learning to exit from the building when the alarm sounded. Instead, they were learning that the alarm was a signal for them to sit and wait until a staff member came to pull them to their feet; they were also learning habits of dropping to the floor or reversing direction in response to physical prompts. These effects were an ironic contrast to the effects intended by the author when he had helped to develop the behavioral plan. Instead of spending the time and the staff meetings that would be necessary to devise a complicated revision of the plan, the author decided to experiment with and develop a procedure in which the hypnotic principles of pacing, leading, and distraction could be applied to more rapidly bring about the learning required.

He asked that the alarm be turned on and he replaced a staff member's position as the prompter for a resident. When the alarm began to sound, he gently but immediately pushed the resident to his feet and gave him a push which propelled him a few steps forward. This was a leading maneuver. As long as the resident continued in the desired direction, without delay, the author did not interfere. If the resident turned from the desired direction, the author paced the move rather than resist it. He did this by taking hold of the resident's arm and following the turn. However, the author continued the turning motion, using the resident's momentum, thus diverting and leading the resident in a complete revolution which again oriented him in the desired direction.

The author also gently prodded and tugged at the resident's arms, hands, and back, which provided a distracting function since the resident could not be sure which prod or tug to oppose. The resident would then be propelled forward by a leading maneuver when caught unawares, unsure of whether the move forward was his own doing or that of the author's and therefore more likely to continue onward in the desired direction. When the resident let his knees buckle, in order to drop to the floor, the author immediately pushed the resident downward, rather than pulling him to his feet. Again, this paced the resident's movement and momentum, going with, rather than opposing, the resident, until the resident opposed this by standing up. If the resident dropped to the floor too quickly for the author to respond in this way, the author accomplished the above maneuver by playfully "bouncing" the resident up and down, rather than simply pulling him to his feet. This confused the resident as to whether he wanted to be on or off his feet and at any point that he chose to stand and walk, the author let go of him.

This procedure produced a very rapid exit from the building. Prompts were withdrawn whenever the resident was performing in the desired direction, with the goal of eventually withdrawing all prompts. The process of pacing, leading, and distraction were explained to staff members and demonstrated until they were understood. The staff then took over the task once again, but with a renewed interest in developing these new skills. The training sessions were now rapid, relatively painless for both residents and staff, and fun.

Case 3: Impotence

Mr. and Mrs. E. had become involved in therapy for problems concerning their daughter. As these problems were in the process of resolution, marital difficulties were revealed which Mr. and Mrs. E. desired to address. One of these consisted of the problem of secondary impotence. This problem had a recent onset and seemed associated with other difficulties in the relationship. Yet, as these other difficulties improved, the problem of impotence remained. Whenever Mr. and Mrs. E. attempted to have sexual intercourse, Mr. E. would either fail to develop an erection or, if having developed an erection, would be unable to maintain it until intromission.

Detailed questioning about the problem revealed a scenario which closely conformed to Masters and Johnson's (1966; 1970) description of secondary impotence. The first occasion on which the problem occurred was one in which Mr. E. was intoxicated. Although he was able to attribute the impotence to the effects of alcohol, he nevertheless considered it a threat to his masculinity. Therefore, although he developed an erection on the next sexual occasion, he became anxious about his ability to maintain the erection; due to this "performance anxiety" and the "spectator role" he was assuming (in which he was focused on how well he was performing), he probably was not receptive to the stimulation that would have maintained his arousal and, as a result, lost his erection. In this way, his anxiety problem only made the problem worse, rendering him impotent with ever greater frequency.

Mrs. E. was understanding, patient, and did her best to arouse him to the point of an erection; however, these responses on her part did not help because they made him feel "less of a man." Despite the fact that Mrs. E. became sexually aroused with ease and enjoyed sex thoroughly, she felt that perhaps she might in some way be inadequate as a woman for failing to arouse Mr. E. As a consequence of these various factors in the situation, they both began to avoid sexual encounters. When sexual encounters did occur, Mr. and Mrs. E. both felt quite pressured to succeed and the outcomes were unfavorable.

The therapist discussed a number of the above facts, gave some advice, and provided instructions for "sensate focus" exercises (Masters & Johnson, 1970); these exercises are intended to help people to discover ways of pleasuring one another without feeling pressured to have intercourse. Mr. and Mrs. E. engaged in these exercises, but failed to follow the rule which prohibited attempts at intercourse. Whenever Mr. E.'s penis became semi-erect, he would attempt to proceed to intercourse. As the degree of intimacy escalated, Mr. E. would lose his erection and Mrs. E. would unsuccessfully try to help him regain it. They were bitterly disappointed by these experiences.

The therapist emphasized that the failures were not due to sexual inadequacy but rather were due to their failure to comply with the instructions. Rigid adherence to the instructions was emphasized for the next week. However, during the next week, the instructions were again violated. While doing the sensate focus exercises, they both became highly aroused and Mr. E., eager to meet his wife's needs and urgent to prove his masculinity, again attempted intercourse. He lost his erection despite Mrs. E.'s valiant efforts to help him sustain it.

Although Mrs. E.'s arousal spurred on Mr. E. to attempt intercourse, the therapist suspected that Mrs. E.'s sexual overtures and initiatives tended to frighten Mr. E., making him fear that her sexuality would overwhelm him and that he could never again measure up to her expectations. The therapist also suspected that Mr. E.'s impotence might be metaphorical for his feeling less powerful relative to Mrs. E. in nonsexual aspects of the marital relationship such as in regard to management of the children or Mrs. E.'s increasing independence.

According to this view of marital problems (Madanes, 1981), a power balance can be restored when the less powerful spouse develops a symptom. Even if the impotence was not metaphorical for other problems in the relationship (which were being addressed in other ways in the therapy), the therapist found it useful to view the symptom of impotence as an unfortunate way of maintaining a power balance. It does this by simultaneously establishing two incongruous hierarchies or power relationships: in an overt and graphic manner, the symptom of impotence put Mr. E. in a less powerful and one-down position in the relationship to Mrs. E.; yet, on a covert level, the symptom's power to persist put Mr. E. in a one-up position and Mrs. E. in a helpless role because try what she might she was unable to arouse him.

This is not to say that Mr. E. was making a conscious effort to remain impotent. An erection is an involuntary response and cannot be commanded to occur. In fact, the voluntary and conscious efforts by both Mr. and Mrs. E. to produce an erection were serving to prevent it. It was necessary to block their usual voluntary behaviors and give them new ones in which to engage. The therapist had also learned by now that the couple could be counted on to follow instructions to the point that an erection was achieved, but could be counted on to disobey the instructions to the extent that Mr. E. would proceed to intercourse and Mrs. E. would do whatever she believed would help him maintain his erection.

The therapist needed to devise an intervention which would capitalize on the constellation of personal and interpersonal factors described above. Therefore, he told Mr. and Mrs. E. that they obviously could not follow instructions properly in performing the sensate focus exercises and that drastic measures were required. He told them he could give them a game to play that could solve their problem, but that they would have to agree to play by the rules and follow the rules to the letter, no matter how odd and unusual the game sounded to them. This was a therapeutic, or hypnotic, suggestion, which conveyed the message that if a ritual is performed properly, positive change will occur. Although no serious attempt had been made to induce a trance, the couple's attention was riveted by what the therapist had said about the need for drastic measures and they were both enthusiastic in their agreement to do whatever was asked of them. The therapist repeated the suggestion that by playing the prescribed game, the problem would subside. Then he prescribed the game.

Instead of the sensate focus exercise, Mrs. E. was to lay flat on her back on a bed, with her hands at her sides, immobile and impassive, like a corpse. It was stressed that she should keep her hands at her sides and make no overtures and take no initiatives, despite anything Mr. E. did to her and despite how aroused she became. She would lose the game by showing too many signs of arousal, which might be a difficult judgement to make, but she would instantly lose it by taking her hands from her sides or engaging in any voluntary sexual behaviors. Mr. E.'s task was to caress Mrs. E. and use any skills he could to try to arouse and please her, perhaps in innovative ways, using either his hands, his mouth, or even his flaccid penis. He did not have to become erect to win the game.

The therapist privately assumed that Mrs. E.'s sexual arousal would be stimulating to Mr. E., but that sexual initiatives on her part would have an opposite effect. Therefore, Mrs. E. was told that she might squirm or display other signs of arousal, but that this was something that she would not be able to help because arousal was an involuntary response; keeping her arms at her sides and laying flat on the bed were voluntary actions, were within her control, and could be accomplished.

The therapist's comments contained the assumption, and therefore the suggestion, that Mrs. E. would become aroused. Even if this suggestion had not been made, the therapist had almost no doubt in his mind that

Mrs. E. would become aroused and display signs of this, despite instructions to remain immobile and to take no action. Yet, the instructions to
remain immobile "like a corpse" were rigid enough to prevent her from
making overtures or taking initiatives which could frighten Mr. E. or
which could be construed as intentional efforts to arouse him.

This prohibition would interrupt or block the usual sequence of interactions consisting of Mr. E. becoming erect, Mrs. E. responding to the
erection with certain voluntary behaviors, Mr. E. beginning to lose his
erection and Mrs. E. trying to help him regain it. Instead, when Mr. E.
became erect he would feel free to lose and regain the erection as often
as he liked without the erection having an interpersonal meaning or
constituting a signal for action by Mrs. E. Her signs of arousal, which
she could not control, would now be construed as evidence of his sexual
mastery and therefore serve to arouse him.

Mrs. E. was told to continue to behave like a corpse even if Mr. E.
became erect. It was stressed that this meant that her arms were to remain
at her sides despite how aroused either of them might become and even
during the intercourse they might have. Mr. E. was to be the one to
decide when the game was over. These instructions contained the implicit
suggestion that erection could occur and that intercourse was permissible.
Yet, if neither erection nor intercourse occurred, Mr. E could still be a
winner and the therapist could be blamed for having given a poor prescription.

When the task was attempted during the next week, Mr. and Mrs. E.
both became quite aroused and Mr. E. was able to maintain an erection
throughout intercourse to the point of orgasm. He regained so much
confidence in his masculinity that he refused to engage in the task again
that week as had been prescribed, and instead resumed a more natural
form of sexual interaction with his wife.

Several hypnotic, strategic, and interactional aspects of this task require
further discussion. First, the task itself contained implicit suggestions for
change, aside from the therapist's suggestions. Any particular suggestions
made by the therapist, while not absolutely necessary to the intervention,
were given to assure that the instructions were clear enough for the task
itself to effectively communicate its implicit demands during the actual
performance of it. For example, one suggestion implied by the task
demands was that Mrs. E. would not be able to stop herself from becoming
aroused. The entire intervention (including both the task and the therapist's instructions) conveyed to the couple a very general but potent
suggestion to give up all direct attempts to produce an erection because

if they followed the rules of the game this desired result would be accomplished on its own.

A message was also conveyed that when an erection did occur, it was permissible to engage in intercourse. This gave Mr. E. permission to do what he was likely to attempt anyway, but the attempt would now be made in an interpersonal context which would permit him to maintain the erection.

Aside from the above suggestions, the task served to indirectly redefine the problem. From a strategic point of view, it is sometimes useful to redefine a problem which consists of an involuntary response or a feeling to a problem which consists of a behavior within the client's voluntary control (Madanes, 1981). In this case, the problem was redefined by redefining the couple's goals.

Mr. E's goal had been to produce an erection. He had been in a relationship with his penis in which he was virtually commanding it to perform, focusing his attention on this goal to a degree that rendered him unreceptive to erotic stimulation. Rather than having the goal of developing an erection, which is an involuntary act and difficult to achieve, the goal was changed to that of using his sexual skills to arouse Mrs. E., skills which were under his voluntary control. Rather than Mrs. E. having to engage in various actions which would stimulate Mr. E., a goal she was unable to accomplish, her goal became that of engaging in the behavior of keeping her arms at her sides, which she could easily accomplish. Yet, she was free to experience sexual arousal as long as she did not act on this with initiatives to arouse Mr. E.

The task also altered the interactional pattern by transforming the interpersonal meaning of, and use of, sexual arousal in the relationship. Rather than Mrs. E. being in a more powerful, one-up position by virtue of her nonsymptomatic status, namely, her sexual arousability, her arousal would now make her a "loser." With Mrs. E's arousal a virtual certainty, any signs of arousal could be construed as evidence of Mr. E.'s triumph; any actions he had taken to arouse her would now be construed as characteristic of his sexual mastery. This would help him to feel more confident in his ability to perform. Because he could pleasure his wife and beat her at this game even with a flaccid penis, there was no pressure on him to develop an erection. While he could be more powerful than Mrs. E. in this respect, his symptom of impotence had lost its power in the relationship. It could no longer be construed as a symptom which Mrs. E. was powerless to affect, since she was told to take no voluntary action to help him to achieve an erection.

This task was admittedly a sexist one, requiring the female to play an impassive role and to be viewed as a "loser" as a result of signs of sexual arousal. However, the task was intended as a temporary measure, not as a prescription for a permanent sexual relationship. The couple could quickly discard it once it had accomplished its purpose. It has been used successfully in another case as well (O'Connor, 1985), with slight variations necessitated by the unique features of the case.

Case 4: The Chores of Life

Many people complain that they are spending too much of their time meeting obligations or engaging in chores which bore them. In some cases, individuals are rushing around and feel overstressed; in others, they have established so many goals that the pleasure they once obtained from the process of meeting those goals is no longer present; and in others yet, they feel that the activities which fill their daily lives are boring or not meaningful. For a variety of these problems, a particular intervention containing only a few suggestions has proved of some value. It results in a redistribution of attention which in turn results in a more interesting experience, whether that experience consists of waiting for a bus or washing dishes. Although it will be illustrated here in the case of Mr. and Mrs. H., it has been used in individual therapy, family therapy, and even on streets or in hallways in casual conversations, with acquaintances and colleagues as well as with clients.

Mr. and Mrs. H. were in therapy for problems concerning their child and their marriage. These were being addressed effectively with a combination of behavioral, strategic, and structural approaches. At one point, Mr. and Mrs. H. both complained about how "burnt out" they felt with all the chores and obligations which consumed their lives. They felt they could not manage to find enough time for the things that were of value. Prioritizing had not helped because none of their chores were dispensible. They apologized for sounding like childish complainers, yet wondered if there was anything the therapist could do to help with this. They doubted that there was anything he could do, pointing out that they were afflicted with the normal and inevitable boredom and stresses of everyday life. They said that they would probably just have to learn to grow up.

The therapist responded by saying that they might be able to find a way to help themselves. He said that their problem was that they were engaging in particular chores as if the chores constituted intermissions from living. For example, they acted as if life stopped when they began to iron a shirt and would begin again when the shirt was ironed. Their attention was on other things, not on ironing the shirt, and they tried to rush through the chore so they could begin living again, thinking only of the odious aspects of the chore. Mr. and Mrs. H. readily agreed, by nods and brief comments, that this was the way they felt.

It was pointed out that they had forgotten that each chore, such as ironing a shirt or washing dishes, was not in intermission from living, but was itself the living of their lives, just as listening to the therapist's voice at that very moment constituted the living of their lives. If they continued to forget this, they could go on wasting chunks of their lives. But if they could remember that each moment of a chore was a part of the living of their lives, then they could make the most of it because their attention would be on it, and they would interact differently with the chore and would notice things about the chore and about living that they were not accustomed to noticing. They were told that if they viewed a chore in this way, they would be involved in a kind of trance because this was a very meditative way of interacting with and engaging in the tasks of living; and that each chore could be viewed as an opportunity to engage in this form of meditation.

They responded with some enthusiasm, saying that they could see how this could be done, and that they looked forward to trying it. However, the therapist cautioned that they could easily forget to view things in this way. He suggested that there was a way for them to automatically enter into this hypnotic manner of interacting with a chore. They could do so by telling themselves, as they began a chore, to "Do it more slowly than usual"; or, if they forgot to do this and found themselves by force of habit in the midst of a chore and feeling rushed and hating the activity, they could instantly alter the experience by saying to themselves "Slow down." They were told that by forcing themselves to reduce their usual pace and slowing their every movement, their attention automatically would become focused on each movement and on each moment. Slowing down would pull them out of their ordinary frame of thought and into the more meditative one which they preferred. In this way, they were told, the injunction to slow down was similar to a post-hypnotic suggestion which would trigger a nonordinary experience.

They were also told that success at this did not depend on meditative ability to go into a trance because the trance induction would occur easily and on its own. Instead, success depended on remembering to force themselves to slow down their movements. They were assured that they need not worry about chores being left undone due to the slower pace; while it might take a little more time to perform a chore or run an errand in this way, the extra time required was actually quite negligible, and the feeling of living life meaningfully, with less anxiety, and less fatigue would enable them to retain the endurance to get much more accomplished.

Since they were interested in Zen Buddhism, they were told that this lesson might be one conveyed by an old Zen koan in which a disciple asked a master for the answer to finding enlightenment. The master answered the disciple by asking if the disciple had washed his pots and pans. It was suggested that washing pots and pans could be more important than ordinarily realized.

Mr. and Mrs. H. immediately commented on several situations in which they believed this method would be helpful. Mr. H. reported subsequently that when he used this method, he was startled at the ease with which he went into a meditative state. He was also surprised by the fact that he enjoyed performing the chore. However, it is not known how often he or Mrs. H. used this method nor whether it became integrated into their general styles of functioning.

Each time this intervention has been applied, the introductory statements describing the person's usual way of thinking (e.g., thinking of chores as odious intermissions from living) establishes an empathic connection and serves to pace the person's experience of the problem. The notion that the chore is itself part of living is an unusual notion and usually rivets attention enough to produce the equivalent of a light trance. It is a notion that the person easily realizes even if not having previously realized it. The act of contemplating this notion can by itself produce the trance-like experience of noticing each movement and each moment.

If it does not, especially in those who tend to intellectualize the notion, the therapist can facilitate it by asking that the person notice how it can happen in the present as he listens to the therapist's voice or glances about the room. The notion that living consists of each moment is one that makes this experience more meaningful, but it is not by itself responsible for the perception of being in a trance or meditation. This perception is due to the redistribution of attention which occurs when a person slows down. Attention is placed on positive aspects as well as odious aspects of the experience, with less attentional capacity available for anticipation of a future activity in which one might wish to be engaged instead.

Case 5: A Therapeutic Mistake

Ms. I. had become involved in therapy to seek help in extricating
herself from a long term relationship with a lover. The therapist took
steps to address this problem with her but noticed that she also complained
repeatedly about how "burnt out" she felt on her job and how overwhelmed she felt by the typing and paperwork which she had come to
dread. She seemed almost to be asking for help with this but switched
topics rapidly whenever the therapist gave it the kind of full attention
that conveyed the message that this problem could be addressed if she
wished to address it. The therapist did not at the time fully appreciate
that Ms. I. did not really wish to focus her energy on solving this problem.
Perhaps she used it as something to complain about when her anxiety,
anger, and sense of loss regarding her lover became too intense to continue
to discuss. Perhaps she did wish to address it, but had energy enough to
address only the most pressing of her problems. The possibilities are
several.

On one occasion in which Ms. I. was complaining about her typing,
the therapist attempted to apply the intervention described in the previous
case example, showing Ms. I. how she could use typing and paperwork
as opportunities to meditate and to enjoy her daily life. When she understood what the therapist was getting at, she did not respond with the
sense of surprise that usually occurs. Yet she did respond with interest
and this response seduced the therapist to continue the intervention. Due
to her interest in oriental philosophy and mysticism, he even illustrated
and "punched up" the intervention with a Taoist verse (about the value
of doing less each day), a shaman's advice (about the value of each
moment), a story about a Zen master (whose ideal was to experience
nirvana during the tasks of everyday life rather than only during deep
meditation), a jewish myth about the "Lamed Vov" (thirty six righteous
people who lived very ordinary lives, upon whom the existence of the
world depends), and a description of a Buddhist form of meditation which
requires concentration on each movement one makes.

Throughout all of this, Ms. I. made occasional comments about how
difficult it would be to apply the method for one or another reason. She
also nodded her head frequently, indicating agreement with the therapist's
ideas, but displayed on her face a sheepish, hangdog expression, as if
to say: "Yes, it's a really good idea and I should try it and I'm probably
very naughty and foolish for not doing so."

It was only after the therapist had finished that he realized he had felt, as he talked, an ongoing need to persuade Ms. I. of the value of this intervention and that he had said far too much. The intervention, as well as the stories, had been wasted, as had the time it had taken to communicate them. The effective ingredient in this intervention occurs in the therapist's discussion of how each chore can be experienced differently by focusing on each moment of it, even focusing on moments in the present, such as on what the therapist is saying and doing. Ms. I. had responded with a ready nod, indicating intellectual understanding and agreement; but these responses also suggested that she was not very absorbed or struck by the concept to respond usefully to it.

In *The Art of War*, Sun Tsu provided advice that is relevant to situations of this kind. In discussing attacks by fire, he pointed out that when a fire is started in the enemy camp but the enemy's troops remain calm, it is wise to bide one's time and not attack. In the present case, Ms. I. remained too calm in the face of the fire the therapist thought he had started. The therapist failed to respond appropriately to this behavior, yet was affected by it and responded inappropriately by attempting to convince her. The factor which appears most responsible for the failure was the symmetrical relationship which the therapist allowed to be established between himself and Ms. I. Her hangdog expression, her intellectualizing of the intervention, her occasional objections to its feasibility, were all expressions of doubt or nonacceptance and as such they could be described as symmetrical maneuvers.

The therapist failed to "go with the resistance" and respond with metacomplementary maneuvers which would have enabled him to stay in charge of who defined the relationship. Instead, the therapist responded to Ms. I. by trying to break down her resistance and convince her into experiencing the hypnotic and therapeutic response. This was not helpful to Ms. I. If a hypnotic relationship could not be established, it would have been just as well to have let the matter drop and either wait until Ms. I. was truly interested in addressing this problem or until Ms. I. found ways to solve or live with the problem on her own, which she may have wished to do.

The case is typical of many in which therapists too eagerly try to be helpful and, by their eagerness, defeat their own purposes. When symmetrical relationships are established, it is very difficult, if not impossible, to bring about positive therapeutic change or hypnotic effects. To do so requires altering the relationship, either subtlety or forcibly, to a complementary one or to one in which the therapist is keeping it unclear to the client whether the client's responses are symmetrical or complementary. It is necessary to take the time to ensure that these kinds of therapeutic relationships exist, rather than a symmetrical relationship. They constitute a basic prerequisite for therapeutic change despite how ingenious or sophisticated any subsequent advice or technique might be. Interventions cannot take hold if the therapist has no leverage or foothold or if the client is not ready to listen. Fortunately, in this case, Ms. I.'s burnout problem was a minor one relative to her other problems and it was only in regard to this problem that a symmetrical relationship existed between herself and the therapist.

Case 6: Relationship Hopping

Everett E. was 30 years of age when he contacted the author with the complaint that he was in the process of inadvertently destroying his relationship with the man with whom he currently lived. It is noted here that Everett's sexual preference was homosexual. He had come to realize that he had been establishing and ruining one relationship after another for over ten years and he wanted to interrupt this pattern. He was motivated to do so at this point because he could see that the man with whom he was presently involved, who will be called Paul, could not be blamed for the deterioration of the relationship (unlike others with whom Everett had been involved in the past). The pain that this deterioration occasioned for Paul had convinced Everett that he had a problem. In addition, Everett was developing a romantic interest with someone else, who will be called Steve, and Everett wanted help in deciding whether to pursue that interest or whether to give it up and try to restore his relationship with Paul.

Although each of his past series of relationships were different, there were certain common features to most of them. Each began with a romantic stage in which Everett charmed the other person and thrived on the other's admiration of him. This romantic period lasted anywhere from three months to something over a year. Then Everett would lose interest and become intolerant of objectionable traits and behaviors in the other which had been overlooked when the other had been on a pedestal. This "cooling off" seemed to occur at a point at which the routines of living together became established and predictable, which made Everett feel as if there were "no way out" and that the other had become too dependent on him. Everett could be characterized as a distancer in these relationships and his partners could be characterized as pursuers who were somewhat possessive and easily aroused to jealousy.

After his partners had been taken off a pedestal, Everett began to pick at them with criticism, go out on one-night stands, and engage in passive aggressive behavior which was designed on a preconscious level to drive the other out of the relationship. Since he engaged in these types of behavior in relation to the other, rather than simply terminate the relationship, the relationship usually suffered a slow and painful death, with this stage of deterioration lasting sometimes as long as a year. This seemed to be due to his unwillingness to take responsibility for termination of the relationship. The relationship usually came to an end when either of them had finally had enough; also, termination was often associated with Everett's development of a new romantic interest, as seemed to be occurring now.

A piece of relevant history, in both Everett's and the author's view, was that he had been closely attached to and identified with his mother, who had died as Everett was entering adolescence. She had held the family together as the only person who could maintain close relationships with everyone. When she died, Everett had assumed the maternal role in his family, but at this stage of early adolescence he was not yet equipped to adequately fulfill it, especially in regard to a capacity for intimate relationships. Overburdened with a role he could not fulfill, he watched helplessly as his family fell apart. He quickly abandoned this role of nurturance and dependability, and instead relied on his charm and impulsivity to insulate himself from pain in a continual spree of acting out behavior during the majority of his adolescence. By his early twenties, he had settled down to a responsible career and resumed a degree of dependability which he believed to be worthwhile in his development. He was distressed by the facts that he repeatedly failed to maintain relationships and that his behavior became undependable towards the end of each relationship.

He was now asking for help in improving his functioning in relationships so that each relationship would not follow the same pattern. He also could not decide what to do now, in regard to either Paul or Steve. When he thought about abandoning Paul and beginning a relationship with Steve he felt tortured by the pain he was causing Paul and worried that he was repeating a cycle; when he thought about staying with Paul he felt hemmed in and deprived. As he struggled to make the right decision, he continued his passive aggressive style with Paul, and his feelings of deprivation and suffocation made Steve appear more appealing. That is, it looked as if the cycle was about to be repeated.

Everett expected that therapy might consist of an exploration of his feelings and of his past and that by this means he might be helped to make the right decision. Yet, the author pointed out that by the time this was done, he might already be involved in a relationship with Steve if the course of events continued to drift as they had seemed to be doing. From Everett's description of his relationship with Paul and from answers he gave to certain questions, the relationship appeared to the author to have deteriorated beyond the point of a recovery; Everett's wish to restore it seemed to reflect more of a concern with Paul's pain than a wish to stay with him. Yet, the author could not be sure.

In the first session, the author suggested to Everett that effective treatment could consist of two main tasks during a preliminary stage and then some other tasks and other therapeutic work at an intermediate stage. These would be explained fully at the next session because there was only time enough remaining in this first session to give Everett the first task. He seemed agreeable to this plan.

The first task consisted of asking him to feel free to go right ahead and to make a bad decision about his life situation rather than waiting until he could figure out the right decision. The task is derived from the interventions developed by the MRI group for the problem of "mastering feared events by postponing them". The rationale is that problems are maintained by avoiding something out of fear of behaving imperfectly. When someone is encouraged instead to approach the avoided event with deliberate intent to negotiate it in an imperfect manner, the person may negotiate the event successfully enough and discover the fear to have been unjustified.

This intervention was applied by suggesting to Everett that "right" decisions do not usually get made by conscious and logical reasoning. He was told that it is possible to make decisions in this way, but not always possible to live with them. Examples were used to illustrate to Everett that we delude ourselves when we believe we have intellectually decided something. Instead, it was suggested that rather than force ourselves to formulate decisions, what we really do is discover what appears to be the best thing to do and then we label it as a decision and come up with many good reasons to support it. A way to help oneself to discover a decision was to go ahead and consciously make a bad decision.

If in trying to live with this decision, one found it appeared best, then one was fortunate to have discovered the right decision at the outset. If the decision had unfortunate consequences, one was still free to make further bad decisions that might reverse the first one. By making bad decisions and beginning to live with them, one can discover what one wants in ways that are not possible with intellectual reasoning alone. The only drawbacks are that others may take action in regard to a bad decision that makes the decision irreversible, and that a bad decision or series of them might be hurtful and confusing to others. These were risks one had to be fully willing to take in following this approach.

Therefore, in announcing his bad decision to those who needed to know it, Everett was asked to inform them that he recognized it was probably a bad decision. He was also to add that he might very well change his mind and make some other decision, and that he was offering his apologies in advance for any confusion or hurt he caused by his decisions. He could also say that others were free to act in any way they thought best in response to his decisions and he too would have to accept those consequences. It was emphasized that it was important that he make announcements of this kind rather than make decisions and express feelings in disguised and passive aggressive ways.

Throughout the above monologue, the messages were conveyed repeatedly that Everett was to stop trying to make the right decision and that the right decision would be made on its own without consicous deliberation. This bi-level, paradoxical message was made all the more plausible because he was given a concrete way to stop trying to make the right decision (by being asked to make bad decisions) and because he was given a concrete understanding of how change would occur automatically (that is, by discovering that a decision has been made involuntarily). By communicating this bi-level message, the author was establishing a hypnotic relationship which was maintained in regard to this as well as subsequent interventions and tasks.

At the completion of these instructions, Everett expressed a sense of freedom and relief, saying that it was nice to have "permission" to make bad decisions. He said, jokingly, that he thought he could be good at it. He was also pleasantly surprised that working out his problems could be accomplished without a painful struggle.

Before leaving, Everett was told that the second task to be given in this preliminary stage was intended to affect his relationship with either Paul or Steve, and would have to await the completion of some bad decisions he made throughout the week because the author could not know where to focus this next task until some decisions had been made. However, Everett was told that if he should decide to leave Paul, it would be best for him to leave his relationship with Steve in exactly the same status as it was now for a temporary period. That is, he should not in any way alter the relationship with Steve, either by accelerating it or terminating it, until he returned to the next meeting.

In the next meeting he described how he made the "bad" decision of leaving Paul and how he had announced it. Though he had done it gently, he had done it directly. He described this as different from his usual passive aggressive approach; he experienced it as more immediately painful than his usual approach but more honest and constructive. Plans were now underway for separation and he and Steve were keeping their relationship "on hold," contacts between them remaining at the same frequency and intensity as previously.

Aside from mourning the loss of Paul, Everett was now worried that if he entered into a relationship with Steve, he would succeed only in causing them both a great deal of pain, and he wondered whether he should try to avoid progressing with this relationship. The author asked if preventing the development of this relationship by trying to avoid it was a realistic possibility. Everett laughed and said no. The author told him that the next task was intended to alter this relationship by either destroying it much more rapidly than was usual or by enriching it in a way that also was not usual for him.

Basically the task consisted of attempting to become an imperfect relationship partner, because he had tried so hard in the past to be a good relationship partner that these noble efforts themselves had created a problem. He was told that he needed a way to stop trying so hard to manufacture a good relationship (which was a message of "stop trying to consciously change") and that if he could stop, then he would discover that a good relationship could develop on its own (which was a message that change could occur). By engaging in a specific task, he could make it more likely to occur on its own (which conveyed the message that change would occur) and at the same time avoid his previously futile efforts to change (which was a message that he should stop trying so hard in his usual ways to change). The specific task is described below.

The author explained to Everett that over the years he had become too charming for his own good. That is, he had overdeveloped his ability to charm a partner in an effort to make a relationship work and the admiration in which he had basked during the first year of any relationship had reinforced a belief that this was the proper way to do it. What had enabled him to be so charming was that he had tried so hard to, or developed a skilled habit of, overlooking characteristics in the other which disqualified the other as a permanent partner in Everett's eyes. These characteristics could be psychologically meaningful (such as possessiveness) or superficial (such as "big ears"). What was important about them was that they allowed Everett to know in advance that he had already written this person off as a permanent partner.

These characteristics could easily be overlooked during the first blush of a romantic relationship, and were likely to be more efficiently overlooked by someone who had perfected good skills to charm others. The high tolerance for objectionable characteristics helped to craft a honeymoon reality. However, it was only later that these characteristics would make their importance felt by engendering conflict. Sometimes these characteristics would constitute the content of a conflict, but other times, the articulation of the characteristics (such as "big ears" which the other could hardly be blamed for) would be so insulting that it would continue to be avoided and the conflict would be displaced onto something else as a screen for the real problem.

A way to identify these characteristics early in a relationship was to notice that it was difficult to admit to even oneself that a particular characteristic in the other was objectionable and to notice how difficult it was to imagine articulating it to the other due to fear of profoundly insulting the other. It was more important to become fully conscious of these pre-conscious perceptions and thoughts than to announce them, but Everett was also asked to announce them. However, he was to be discriminating and to announce only the characteristics which were devastating; since none of these were intolerable to him in the honeymoon period, he could double check on whether it was truly a significant characteristic by viewing it from the point of view of the deterioration stage in a time projection into the future.

He was told that this was not an instruction for his insides to become visible to the other or for him to become ruthlessly honest about every little thing that bothered him about the other. In addition to distorting the interaction in a maladaptive way, ruthless honesty of this kind was needlessly hurtful and not good manners. If he was discriminating, then his announcements would be few but powerful. They would either bring the relationship to a much more rapid end, which would be a merciful act to his partner, or would enrich it by increasing the range of interaction that was possible, and thereby make it more realistically painful, rather than magically euphoric. Everett was asked to explain his task to Steve so that Steve would be aware of the fact that this relationship was an experiment in altering a pattern and could make his own decision as to whether he wished to remain or leave.

The author expected that Everett would also attempt to charm the author; the author had already experienced the countertransferential response of feeling charmed. Instead of waiting for Everett to cool off to the author to point out the transference, the author now explained his expectations and asked that Everett keep himself honest in his task with Steve by using the author to practice his task. He could do this by noticing traits and behaviors and habits of speech in the author he found to be objectionable but which were easy to overlook early in the relationship. In this way, the issue of transference could be openly and easily addressed from the outset and could reinforce the strategic and hypnotic interventions which were underway.

It is difficult to discriminate objectionable characteristics in another which one would prefer not to acknowledge to even oneself and which one often does so only at a preconscious level. Therefore, it required much discussion in subsequent sessions to keep alive the importance of this task. It resulted in painful announcements which were unusual for Everett to make in relationships, but not so painful as anticipated, and which in turn resulted in unpredictable and interesting turns of events.

Following this preliminary stage of treatment, the focus turned to Everett's conflict in regard to dependability and undependability and to his tendency to be the "power" in the relationship (or the one to define it). Tasks were assigned in regard to these issues. In addition, time was spent on "working through" conflicts and pain associated with his mother's death in a manner that conformed to a psychodynamic approach. His role in his family of origin was also explored, going back three generations, utilizing concepts and methods derived from a family systems approach developed by Bowen, Fogarty, Guerrin, and others at the Center for Family Learning in New Rochelle, N.Y. The final outcome of Everett's treatment is not yet known.

Case 7: Temper Tantrums

Willie T. was four years of age when Mr. and Mrs. T. contacted the author to ask for help in reducing Willie's temper tantrums. The tantrums had begun approximately six months previous and had steadily gotten worse. Nothing the parents had tried had been effective in reducing them and they sometimes occurred several times a day. They typically occurred in a context in which Willie was being asked to do something, such as brush his teeth or put on his clothes. He would refuse, the parent would repeat the demand and perhaps reason with him, he would argue back with his own reasons and would again refuse, but louder and more rudely. The parent would respond with more reasons or more anger, and these exchanges would continue until Willie began to flail and kick and scream.

Mrs. T. tended to be more empathic and to reason and argue more with him, which tended to draw out the symmetrical escalation prior to the eruption of tantrums; Mr. T. tended to be more demanding and angry and was quicker to force a toothbrush into Willie's mouth. Despite these differences in style, about which the parents argued, the parent-child interaction leading to tantrums was essentially the same. Following a tantrum, Mr. T. would accuse Mrs. T. of being too soft and Mrs. T. would accuse Mr. T. of being too heavyhanded. Although neither parent handled Willie more effectively than the other, it was Mrs. T. who had more reason to complain because Willie was in her care more of the time.

Mr. and Mrs. T. both worked full time and had done so throughout their marriage. Mrs. T. had only taken time off for maternity leave, first with the birth of Willie and then with the birth of Sandra who was now two years of age. When Willie had been born, the responsibilities of having a family became vivid to Mr. T. and he expressed some ambivalence about his commitment to the family. Mrs. T. was hurt by this and resented it, but reacted by taking on more of the child care responsibilities.

Mr. T.'s ambivalence about commitment and Mrs. T.'s resentment were not discussed further, but this marked a point at which some of the warmth and fun in the marital relationship began to wane. With the birth of Sandra, Mrs. T. assumed even more of the child care responsibilities because she didn't feel she could expect an uncommited man to share the burden. The role differentiation that evolved seemed justified in Mr. T.'s view because whenever he had participated in any child care activities he had been criticized by Mrs. T. as not performing them correctly. He concluded that she wanted him out of that area and that she was content with assuming primary responsibility for child care. She, on the other hand, was furious that she had so much responsibility on her shoulders. Yet, neither of them spoke of these matters and were quite unclear as to what the problem was between them.

Willie's tantrums provided an opportunity to at least verbalize a limited portion of their conflict—her being too involved with the children and he being too remote. Aside from these communications and communication about the logistical arrangements of everyday life, the couple did not communicate with one another in ways they had earlier in their marriage. They had not been out alone with one another for years, although this was something they had thoroughly enjoyed before the children had been born.

The problem of temper tantrums had also been associated with some adjustment problems Willie was having in his preschool class, about which he was angry and confused. The author also believed it may have been metaphorical for Mr. T.'s anger with some people in his work setting, or for Mrs. T.'s anger at Mr. T.'s lack of involvement in family life. However, it seemed most likely that it was an overt expression of the unspoken conflict between the parents. It allowed each of them to verbalize the conflict to a limited extent as it pertained to the tantrums. Yet it also distracted them from their inability to adequately address the ominous and silent conflict that had grown between them.

Using Madanes' rationale, the tantrums may have been metaphorical for this parental conflict and may have established a hierarchical incongruity that temporarily restored a power balance between the parents. Each of the parents had felt increasingly threatened in their relationship with one another as their roles became more differentiated over time as a result of misunderstandings. The tantrums distracted them from this problem and brought the parental best out of them; yet, their hierarchical superiority as parents was incongruous with their inability to control the tantrums in their child. "Pretend" strategies were considered by the author in order to resolve the hierarchical incongruity. Some other strategy seemed necessary to restore the balance of power in the relationship between the parents.

From a structural perspective, it was clear that Mrs. T. had developed an overclose relationship with the children and that Mr. T. was somewhat disengaged. His relationship with work and her's with the children and their anger with one another about these facts effectively blocked the warm relationship they had had in the past with one another. In addition, though the mother's relationship with the children remained overclose, it had changed from a predominantly positive one to a more negative one due to the burden it became for her. What seemed necessary was to increase Mr. T.'s closeness with the children, decrease Mrs. T.'s, and open an avenue for enjoyable communication between the parents.

From a behavioral perspective, Willie's defiant behavior was being positively reinforced by each parent whenever either of them reasoned with or argued with him, instead of punishing him. By the time they did institute any punishment they had already repeatedly reinforced a chain of unacceptable behaviors. That is, they were shaping and teaching him to misbehave, and then capping the process with a punishment which,

by the time it was administered, had little effect on the targeted misbe-
havior. What was necessary was to administer potent punishing events
with immediacy and certainty and to block the parents from arguing or
reasoning with the child.

From a family development perspective, the family relationships had
undergone some typical changes with the advent of the children. The
advent of children represents a transition from one stage to another in
family development. It is quite typical for a parent to feel ambivalent
about commitment at this point. Mr. and Mrs. T.'s reactions to this
ambivalence and their solutions for it were also somewhat common, but
were preventing them from successfully negotiating this transition. They
needed to be maneuvered out of this stalemate and back onto the track
of growth and development as a family.

The author provided three distinct interventions in the first session. He
first explained that he had a number of things in mind that could serve
to put them back on track, and that only a few of these would be explained
in this session. The rest would be held in reserve until the effects of the
first few interventions had been monitored. This conveyed a clear message
that whatever the author asked them to do would have the effect of
bringing about desired change.

The author then explained that he assumed that Mr. T. was sufficiently
committed to the family and that in the author's experience some ambivalence about this commitment was normal. He told Mr. and Mrs. T.
that their problem was that they didn't know how to adequately address
this ambivalence and had developed patterns of interaction that implied
a lack of commitment, which the author suggested was a mistaken implication. The author said that instead of talking about commitment, he
would prefer to simply provide a test of Mr. T.'s commitment in an
experiment that would severely tax Mr. T.'s resources, if Mr. T. was
willing to try it. He agreed he was willing. Before explaining the experiment, the author said to Mrs. T. that he realized she did not approve
of Mr. T.'s style of caring for the children, but asked if she thought that
the children would be in any actual danger with him. She replied that
they would not.

He then asked them to simply switch roles for one week, on a temporary
and experimental basis, with Mr. T. taking charge of all child care. Mrs.
T. was to involve herself with the children only to play with them, not
to feed them nor to give them baths or other routines of child care. Mr.
and Mrs. T. both laughed and seemed momentarily stunned by the suggestion, but agreed to it. The author asked if they were sure they would

follow this suggestion and said to them that they shouldn't even begin to try if they couldn't pull it off.

He suggested they now discuss the day to day logistical planning required to reverse roles in this way. He also told Mrs. T. that she was to avoid criticizing Mr. T.'s child care performance or advising him on it no matter how incompetent it might appear to her, but that she was free to laugh at it if she liked. She liked this idea but Mr. T. worried that he might need her advice. He was told he could use her as a consultant for advice, but that he had to ask for the advice; she was not to provide any unsolicited consultation.

From a structural point of view, this role reversal constituted a temporary restructuring of family relationships which, in a stagewise fashion, was preparatory for a final, more optimal restructuring of relationships. From a strategic perspective, it served to block each parent's previous solutions to address their relationship problem by requesting that they each do the opposite of what they had been doing. It will be recalled that this blocking function is equivalent to the message of "Don't change" or "Don't try to lift your arm on purpose."

The intervention was also intended to produce the result achieved in the story of the husband who complained to his rabbi about all the children and in-laws occupying a one room house. The rabbi progressively asked him to bring into the house the goats, then the chickens, then the cow, and so on, with the complaints by the husband getting progressively worse with each new occupant. When the rabbi finally allowed the man to remove all the animals, the man was greatly relieved and profusely thanked the rabbi for helping him. In the present case, the intervention was intended to poise Mr. T. for a more realistic assumption of child care responsibilities.

After Mr. and Mrs. T. had discussed the logistics of the role reversal, the author asked them to stop arguing and reasoning with their son. He explored with them certain punishments that had the promise of potency and he asked them to instantly apply these with no more than one warning. This blocked previous solutions the parents had used to get their son to change and the author was specific in pointing this out to them. He explained that they needed to stop trying to get their son to do what they wanted by arguing and reasoning.

Instead they could teach him responsibility by letting him decide what he wanted to do and learning that he was responsible for the consequences of his decisions. They could let him make his choices and they could simply feel sad when he chose behavior leading to punishment. He needed to do this and they could let him do this without feeling angry, knowing they were helping him. These new rules were explained to Willie and Willie was encouraged to misbehave at home to test out the rules, if he was willing to live with the suffering that these tests would incur. He was also told that sometimes his parents would be unfair, but that they would not argue or reason with him. They would only reason and discuss and listen to his feelings and thoughts later, at quiet times when no one was trying to get him to do something.

Finally, the parents were asked to find a babysitter and to hire her and plan to go out together once a week. Some activities were then explored which they used to enjoy together. They were motivated to hire the babysitter within a week by the author asking them to leave Sandra home with the babysitter during their next appointment.

When they returned a week later, Mr. T. was exhausted and jokingly expressed mock anger towards the author. He said he had learned and realized a great deal throughout the week, but he did not go into any specifics. They reported that Willie's tantrums had been dramatically reduced in frequency, down to about three for the week, all of which were minor in intensity compared to previously.

The author asked the parents to renegotiate the distribution of care-taking responsibilities so that it was a more equitable distribution, and they spent some time doing so. With Mrs. T. prepared to take up some of the slack, Mr. T. was asked to experiment with and discover how he could be more of a playful companion to his son, rather than always teaching him things in a critical and authoritative manner. He found this difficult, not knowing where to begin, but he agreed it was important. The author suggested he begin by ambushing his son with hugs. It was also suggested that Mr. T. might discover ways to have fun with his son in the next task to be assigned.

The author explained that they should not get "too happy" yet, because Willie was still having tantrums and could even relapse back to having many tantrums each day. Therefore, in addition to the new rules for punishing defiant behavior, the author suggested that they engage in certain "pretend" tasks each evening which he said would have an impact on the problem. First he asked Willie and Mrs. T. to show him what usually happened, in an enactment of the problem. After he had seen enough to enable him to coach them, he asked Mrs. T. to ask Willie to pretend to try to get his mother to brush her teeth and for Mrs. T. to pretend to refuse, and to pretend to escalate the conflict to a tantrum. They did so with some coaching and thoroughly enjoyed themselves. Mr.

T. was then asked to engage in the same enactment with Willie, and he did so, utilizing a different content than teeth brushing.

They were then asked to reverse roles, with Willie pretending to be defiant. At one point, where the acting became very loud and convincing and where Willie appeared frightened, the author pointed out to Willie that this was only pretend, not real, and discussed this with him to be sure he understood. The family was asked to perform both pretend tasks each evening and they agreed to do so.

The strategic functions of these pretend tasks have been elaborated in Chapter Ten. Briefly, when the child pretends to have a problem, the fact that it is pretend implies that there is no problem; and when the parent either pretends to have a problem or asks the child to pretend to have the problem, it implies that the parent is really in charge. This transforms the meaning of the problem. The pretended problem can no longer be an expression of parental conflict or a metaphor for a problem in a parent from which the parent is distracted. These functions (and other functions outlined previously) transform a hierarchical incongruity to a single hierarchy, with parents in charge of the child. These tasks also provide an avenue for parents and children to have fun together. The hypnotic functions fulfilled by pretend tasks were pointed out in Chapter Four.

When the family returned the following week, the tantrums had entirely ceased and everyone was functioning in more adaptive ways with one another. No further complaints existed. The parents were seen alone for a part of this session and asked if they were comfortable with the progress and if there was anything else they wished to address. They were told that the author could continue to help them monitor progress and address certain issues, but that it was possible that they felt capable of proceeding on their own and that they might not need the author's help at this point They were also specifically asked if they felt a need to further address any problems between themselves.

They responded by saying that they were doing better at letting each other know what needed to be known and that they thought they were back on track and could handle problems between them on their own. They said that if there were any difficulties between themselves or with Willie which they couldn't handle, they would call, but that they thought they might be ready to try to handle things on their own at this point if the author thought this wise. The author thought it was wise and treatment was terminated. Follow-up calls three and nine months later revealed no further problems that the family could not handle.

Case 8: A Problem of Occupational Identity

Mr. A. was 35 years of age when he and his three daughters began treatment with the author. Mr. A.'s wife had left him a number of years earlier for another man and she no longer had any contact with the family. Mr. A. had been collecting public assistance most of his adult life and had only been employed several times for brief periods. He left these jobs because he either did not like them or could not master them. He did not wish to work because he preferred sleeping late and did not view himself as capable of fulfilling adult responsibilities.

His mood was depressed, his appearance was dishevelled, and he often impressed others as being intellectually "slow" despite the fact that his intelligence was in the average range. He had received previous diagnoses of Depression and Inadequate Personality (according to the DSM II) and had a history, beginning in his childhood, of depending on therapists, social service agencies, and a variety of other helping agents. Most of the helpers involved in his life eventually became frustrated and hopeless, due to Mr. A's failure to benefit from their efforts to help him.

This history was already known when the author became involved in the case as a result of Mr. A. contacting a public mental health agency where the author was on the staff. In speaking to the intake worker, Mr. A. requested help in controlling the misbehaviors of his three unruly daughters. This was a problem that had been addressed numerous times by previous therapists in this and other agencies. However, at the beginning of the first session, when the author asked what the problem was and what Mr. A wanted to see changed, Mr. A. did not specifically mention the problem of controlling his children's behavior. Instead, he replied that the problem was that he was a "loser" and that everything he touched "fell apart." This, then, became the initial problem focus rather than the misbehaviors of the children.

In this and subsequent sessions, Mr. A was seen by the author who had the benefit of a consultation team which was situated behind a one-way mirror. During sessions, the author and the team freely consulted with one another whenever either felt the need to do so.

Towards the end of the first session, the author and the consultants conferred and hypothesized that Mr. A.'s repeated failures in life may have contributed to his depression and poor self image but that in a reciprocal fashion his depression and poor self image had contributed to continuing failures. They also hypothesized that his self image of an incompetent "loser" reflected a need to be very different from his own parents and siblings, who happened to be very competent upper middle class professionals with whom Mr. A. was covertly angry.

Since his parents and siblings had always attempted to help and to improve Mr. A.'s functioning, his enduring incompetence not only served to express separateness and anger in regard to them, but successfully defied their competence. While their competence put them in a more powerful hierarchical position relative to Mr. A., their repeated failures to help him to improve simultaneously allowed Mr. A. to feel one-up on them. Finally, his incompetence provided an excuse to avoid many frustrations and burdens of normal adult life and elicited a great deal of helping behavior from friends, relatives, and helping agents, all of which served to recapitulate Mr. A.'s relationship with his parents.

Even if this formulation was not entirely accurate, it was plausible enough as a rationale to be suggested to Mr. A. in an effort to obtain leverage for interventions which could facilitate change. Rather than ask Mr. A. to follow advice which would improve his functioning in various areas of his life, which all previous helping agents had done, the author told him that there seemed to be a number of advantages in being a "loser." He was told that perhaps the advantages outweighed the disadvantages, and that perhaps it wasn't in his best interest for him to become more competent.

The author went further and suggested that Mr. A. might want to consider learning to become even more artful at being incompetent in order to maximize gains and minimize losses; and if so, the author would try to help him to do so. Mr. A. was disarmed and riveted when he comprehended what the author was communicating to him, but he did not appear to feel insulted, probably due to the author's sincerity and to the rapport that had been established.

This paradoxical approach, which can be considered a derivation of other strategic approaches (e.g., the MRI group's or Madanes'), was sustained over numerous sessions in which various advantages and disadvantages of competence and incompetence were examined and Mr. A. was coached to behave in a more artfully incompetent manner. Over time, nonparadoxical tasks and indirect suggestions which requested specific behaviors were gradually interspersed and when these were completed successfully, more and more of them were assigned. They included tasks which served to improve Mr. A.'s physical appearance and grooming, his physical health and strength, his diet, his manners, his control over his children, his relationship with his extended family, and his development of a social support network unrelated to public agencies.

As the number of straightforward tasks increased, they were often assigned in an interpersonal context which triangulated Mr. A. The triangulation was accomplished by the author taking the position that he believed Mr. A. would complete the task because he was ready for more positive change, and by the consultation team disagreeing with that position because they did not feel that there were sufficient advantages for further improvement. This use of the consultation team is discussed elsewhere and more fully by Papp (1980).

Although strategic and structural models dominated the thinking about this case, it would be a mistake to ignore the other models which were usefully applied. Many of the sessions were individual ones rather than family sessions and therefore a strong transference developed which was addressed not only by the strategic triangulation noted above, but also by analytic interpretation. In addition, since so much of Mr. A.'s behavior was related to his relationships with his family of origin, the therapy entailed the development of a genogram and coaching on interactional behavior with his extended family, typical of extended family systems approaches to therapy.

Despite gradual and continued improvements in various areas of his life, Mr. A. remained ambivalent about improvement. At periodic intervals this conflict was heightened and made overt by the author with the intent to prevent relapses. Due to Mr. A.'s more competent functioning, as well as to circumstances out of his control, he was taken off public assistance against his will and forced to find a job which he found most distasteful. He then faced the choice of continued improvement or rapid deterioration. In the latter event, he anticipated help from a number of sources, including a reinstatement of public assistance.

In the initial days of his new job, he complained a great deal about the details of task demands, as well as complaining about the pressure of holding down a job he did not like while at the same time fulfilling family responsibilities. However, following a three week period in which he became more accustomed to his job, he ceased complaining about specific task demands and complained only about the overall pressure of having to both work and care for his family. Although hypnotic methods had previously and frequently been used with Mr. A., the author utilized these methods again at this point in a manner similar to that illustrated in Chapter Seven with Mrs. B. The purpose was to capitalize on what the author detected to be a slight positive change in Mr. A.'s attitude towards his job, by highlighting this change and suggesting that it could continue to occur. Just prior to the therapeutic suggestions used to accomplish this, Mr.A. and the author had been talking about Mr. A. having effectively punished his daughter Sally for breaking a curfew. A portion of the transcript appears below along with a running commentary.

Transcript

Author: So, Sally's getting over her shock that you mean business when you tell her what to do. She's getting used to it.
Mr. A: Yeah (*laughs*). And it's about time.
Author: I'm glad. But you know, I'd like to get back to something else you were talking about before (*pause*). Something important that you were talking about. (*The author has begun to slow his rate of speech, lower his tone of voice, gradually increase the number of pauses between phrases, unfolds arms, reduces random movements, and maintains as much eye contact as is comfortable for Mr. A*). Something very important.

The author's comment that he wants to talk about something important generates an expectancy that something unusual may be about to occur, analogous to the expectancy of trance in formal inductions. His changes in voice and nonverbal behavior also begin to fixate Mr. A.'s attention.

Mr. A: About what? (*Mr. A. looks puzzled and expectant and reduces random movements*).
Author: About a very serious matter. About this dilemma you are in (*pause*).

The author pauses so that the client may wonder what dilemma is being referred to. This comment may to some extent depotentiate conscious strategies of thought; it should generate an internal search and redistribute attention away from the sensory environment and onto inner experience. The author's next comments will direct or lead the client's attention to the dilemma, which is a conflict with which the client is familiar due to either previous insights by the client or previous persuasion by the author. The subsequent comments serve to pace the client's experience of this conflict.

Author: This dilemma, it's a conflict, between whether you want to be competent or whether you want to be incompetent. You can't decide and you stay on the fence, stuck there, and as you know, it has always been with you, this dilemma, though you only really realize this dilemma once in awhile, how it paralyzes you, keeps you on the fence, keeps you from being competent and keeps you from being totally incompetent. On the one hand, you don't like the stigma of being considered incompetent or abnormal or handicapped. You want to be able to accomplish certain goals and to be successful at these goals like any normal person. And in the past months you've been showing that you can accomplish such goals and have been becoming more and more competent with your daughters, with making friends, with the way you come across to people, with your taste in clothes, with feeling more one-up with your family, and with your assertiveness in general, and now you're holding a job too.

But on the other hand, the price of all this competence is that it puts so much pressure on you and causes hassle after hassle which you'd just as soon avoid, and these pressures make you wish to break down and fail and become incompetent and to let everyone know that you can't be expected to do all those normal things, because then you'd get people to help you out and you could sleep late again and you could show people, like your parents and even me, that no matter how competent they are they aren't good enough to get you to do what they want because you're more competent at being incompetent than they are at making you competent, and you'll show them. Perhaps you would prefer to be competently incompetent than incompetently competent. But, then again, you're not sure it's worth losing all the gains you've made. You sure are in some dilemma. Stuck. Right on the fence.

These reasons and rationales for Mr. A.'s problem (whether they are true or only plausible to his view of the world) are unnecessary to hypnotic work. Yet, since the context is one of ordinary conversation in a typical therapy setting without the use of hypnotic trappings and formal techniques, these rationales are utilized to fulfill certain hypnotic functions. They have paced the client's conflict and have also led the client in the sense that they exaggerate or caricature the conflict in a manner that fixates and rivets attention. The last few sentences have also utilized polarizing terms in close proximity, such as "losing all the gains" and "more competent at being incompetent"; these come close to a literary device which uses antonyms together to describe something, such as "blackest white," or "darkness visible," or "competent incompetence." These were intended to depotentiate conscious sets.

Author: It is the same dilemma you have always been in but there is something different about it this time.

The statement that there is something different this time is also intended to depotentiate conscious sets because the client will wonder what is different but will not be immediately told, and instead will have to focus on what the therapist does say to him.

Author: Of course, this dilemma is not new. It didn't crop up in this room, but you'll end up thinking about this dilemma here, or noticing it, without even trying to. Because it goes back (*pause*). To other phases of your life (*pause*). And is within you (*pause*). And has occured with other people (*pause*). In other jobs you've had (*pause*). In your earlier struggles to function as a single parent (*pause*). And even further back, during your marriage (*pause*). And even further (*pause*) to your childhood (*pause*), when your parents expected so much of you (*pause*). In each phase of your life.

The above comments lead the client to view past experiences with the conflict imposed on those experiences, a different way for this client to remember his past. The pauses allow the client to make links, in his own way, between the author's comments and the client's own idiosyncratic memories. The comments also suggest that he will continue to observe the dilemma without any conscious effort, which facilitates the perception that this experience is involuntary and not effortful. The comments also distract attention from features of the immediate environment. The client's respiration rate and eyeblink reflex were slowed at this point in time, body movement was not observable, and musculature in the face was relaxed.

Author: You've always had this dilemma but there is something different about it this time. What is different is finding that you're enjoying your competence a great deal, for example, your competence with your children, or, as another example, that you're finding that work isn't so bad as it used to be, and you don't hate it as much, nor is it as bad as you thought it would be. And these things are puzzling to you because you figure it doesn't make sense for you to be changing your attitude about work, since you never did before. It puzzles you because it doesn't feel like you. The way you view yourself is on a fence, stuck, in the middle, and not getting too competent. And as you've become more and more competent you haven't really noticed these successes enough to change your view of yourself to that of a more competent individual who is able to handle responsibilities.

The focus of the above comments is on change that is not fully noticed and not yet accommodated by Mr. A.'s self image. Changes which are discrepant with the self image could generate disorientation and anxiety, which could trigger a relapse. Therefore, the author was attempting to account for feelings of disorientation and to catalyze a shift in self image. He then tells a story below, which provides an analogy to the client's situation.

Author: It was the same for me when I first learned to drive a car. I didn't think of myself as a driver of a car. My self image was that of a person who couldn't drive very well. And this was so even after I had my license. I was always trying to keep in mind that the directional was on the left and the gear shift on the right and trying not to confuse the two, and worrying if I would forget whether you shifted gears before you turned the ignition on or whether you turned the ignition on first and whether you put your foot on the brake or on the accelerator when you shifted gears, and I was so worried I might forget what to do next and forget where everything was, that I couldn't very well have the self image of a person who knows exactly how to drive a car. But I kept on doing it, all those little things I had to remember to do, and little by little it became habitual, and soon I didn't have to think about it anymore, and just did all those things automatically, because I had really learned it all, and I didn't know how I did it but everybody does it that way, and I also couldn't tell you exactly when it was that I became a driver and had a self image of a driver, because it happened so gradually, and kind of sneaked up on me. And now that I'm a good driver, I know I couldn't tell you whether the directional is on the left or the right of the steering wheel, because that's not something I have to be conscious of anymore and I can just trust that I automatically will do what's right because I unconsciously know where it is.

The focus of the story was on the difficulties of early learning and on unconscious mastery. Due to this focus, the determination of a change in self image seemed almost tangential. However, the next two stories focus less on difficulties of learning to master a task and more on the issue of how difficult it is to specify when quantitative changes result in a qualitative change in self image. The purpose of this sequence is to create resonance for the latter theme and build on accelerating potency for the theme of alteration of self image.

Author: This is also similar to when I first grew a beard, so many years ago. I've had a beard so long that my self image is that of a bearded person. And when I close my eyes and think of myself, I see myself with a beard. But when did I first have that self image? It's so hard to say. It sneaks up on you. When I first was growing a beard, I first had a little five o'clock shadow, and then a few days later, some stubble, and it was all itchy, but I still thought of myself as a person without a beard. And when I looked in the mirror, I just looked like a grubby sort of person who hadn't shaved in a few days. And it grew and it grew and finally became a full beard and I looked in the mirror each day and said, "Yes, you have a fine beard there," but if I closed my eyes I still thought of myself as a person without a beard. And I can't tell you exactly when, maybe a few weeks, or even a few months, but one day I noticed that I thought of myself as a bearded person and that was my self image from then on.

And that self image grew stronger and stronger with each day and is even growing stronger now. I know that my self image changed little by little, but I hardly noticed it as it happened, but once it happened, I was surprised that it happened, because it had happened almost without me knowing. And it's happening to your daughter Sally. At first, she thought you were just acting weird when you punished her and she was shocked, and then she started getting used to it, and little by little she changed her view of you, and she hardly noticed herself changing her view of you, but her view did change, because now she views you as a parent who means business, thought I bet she couldn't tell you exactly when that view changed, because it's so hard for us to notice such things.

The stories were intended to suggest and to access certain understandings about attitudinal change, so that these understandings would anchor and facilitate the following suggestions.

Author: And the same thing is happening to you. You still have your dilemma, stuck on the fence, but something's different. You feel very puzzled that it's easier to get through the workday, when it used to be so difficult. These mixed feelings about work, both good ones and bad ones, are very puzzling, and you don't like being so puzzled and would like for it all to make more sense. And you know that you've been able many times in the past to discover solutions to such puzzles when you least expected, and even now may be beginning to sense that there is a change in attitude towards work which you will be pleasantly surprised to discover is developing. Attitudes are such curious things. You don't just decide to have a certain attitude, for example, your attitude towards me or towards chocolate ice cream, or towards anything else. You discover suddenly that you have developed one, or are in the process of developing one, and sooner or later, whether it is in an hour from now, or sometime tomorrow, or in a few days, you can discover it, and perhaps feel pleasantly surprised. Do you really understand, I mean, really understand, how your attitude is changing?

The pacing and leading statements contained in the above comments have been identified previously, in an example given in Chapter Three. The last question directs Mr. A.'s attention to whether or not he *really* understands that his attitude is changing, not to whether it is changing. An implied suggestion, or assumption, is made that the attitude is indeed changing, but Mr. A. is distracted from addressing this underlying assumption by the question that asks him to address whether he really understands it is changing. Additional distraction is accomplished by the maneuvers illustrated below which are equivalent to trance termination in formal applications of hypnotic methods.

Author: You know, I keep thinking about Sally's shock at your limit setting. But, you know, I forgot to ask you if she's still improving at school. By the way, how long has it been since she's come to a session here? Three weeks?

The author has animated his voice, has crossed his legs, and has resumed normal interaction similar to that which occurred previous to therapeutic suggestons. The client's attention is directed to topics discussed prior to the suggestions.

Mr. A: Oh, she's been good at school. Getting B's and A's.
Author: When did she last come here?
Mr. A: Oh, about four weeks ago. Maybe five. I'm not sure. (*Bodily movements increase*)

The author continues to ask questions and direct the conversation to usual topics until he is satisfied that Mr. A. is entirely oriented to his current surroundings.

In the next several weeks, the author made no direct inquiries about Mr. A.'s attitude towards work. However, in any work related discussions, Mr. A.'s comments reflected his having noticed slight changes of attitude towards work. Three months later, when becoming dissatisfied with his current job and considering looking for another job, he was able to articulate a definitely altered attitude towards work which reflected a changed self image. This can be best described by his preference to be competitively employed and respected by others rather than be supported by public assistance. About six months later, therapy was terminated. At a one-year follow-up, Mr. A. was happy in a full time job, enjoying a social life, and continuing to behave competently with his children and with other matters.

Case 9: Generalized Anxiety Disorder

Mrs. G. was a single mother in her early forties who called for an appointment concerning the oppositional behavior of her daughter Mary. However, she came alone to the appointment. She said that she had so many problems that she did not know where to begin. She also said that she did not even know if she had any real problems, but that she felt so anxious and upset that she did not know what to do. She talked for awhile about her problems with her daughter Mary; then about harassment from

her ex-husband and how her ex-husband used Mary as a spy to monitor
Mrs. G.'s personal life; then about Mrs. G.'s mother, who intruded upon
Mrs. G.'s relationship with her daughter and who criticized her parenting
practices; then about her automobile, which was always breaking down;
then about her need to lose weight and her feelings of depression; then
about her problems with her boss. She went on and on, from one topic
to another.

In response to questions inquiring what it was she wanted to change
or to work on in therapy, she continued to shift from one problem or
topic to another. Throughout her litany of complaints, she repeatedly
complained of an overwhelming sense of anxiety, dread, and panic.
Although she felt it to be debilitating at those times when she felt overwhelmed by specific problems and stressful situations, she had experienced it on an ongoing basis for over five years. She described her general
style of functioning as "scatterbrained." Specifically, this meant that she
approached every task with a degree of anxiety which interfered with
performing tasks effectively and which also gave her the appearance of
a flustered, incompetent child. The first session ended with the author
feeling unsure of what had been accomplished in the session and feeling
confused about what direction to take.

In the second session, the author again tried to establish a direction
or goal, but Mrs. G. again flitted from one topic to another. The author
hypothesized to himself that Mrs. G. might not really wish to address
her problems in concrete ways, but might instead be the kind of person
who desired from therapy the benefits of a therapeutic relationship, the
opportunity to free-associate and abreact, and a trusted person in whom
to confide. Yet, this remained only a tentative hypothesis because Mrs.
G. continued to request help in regard to specific problems.

It did become more clear that she wanted to learn to deal with the
inevitable stressful situations in life with less anxiety; she spoke several
times of feeling a need for a fundamental change in the way she handled
stress. She also insisted on addressing each of the stresses in her life, yet
would not stick to a discussion of any one of them for long enough for
the author to adequately begin determining how to properly intervene.
Mrs. G. did not know which stress or problem was most important and
she wished for all of them to be addressed at once. She complained of
feeling "crazy" and inadequate for not knowing why she felt so overwhelmed, and wondered whether she was complaining about stress which
was normal and with which others could readily cope.

The author interrupted her, apologizing for his rudeness, and told her that he would have to stop her at this point because she was clearly so overwhelmed that she would be able to go on like this forever, which would not give him an opportunity to see if there was anything that could be done to help her. He went on to point out that she seemed to have two main problems: one was a need to handle stressful situations with less anxiety; the other was a need to figure out which stressful situations were contributing to her anxiety and to then decide which of these she wished to address. He told her that it was clear to him why she felt so overwhelmed at the moment, because anyone would feel overwhelmed if they were embedded in the constellation of stresses that she had described.

He told her that it could help her if this constellation of stresses were clearly identified. She would then know exactly what the sources were of her anxiety and could decide which source she preferred to address first. She could then decide which ones she might prefer to address on her own and which ones she could use the therapist for. It was suggested to her that if she did not know what these sources of anxiety were, she might be anxious in a situation that was not truly anxiety-provoking, and yet, because she was anxious there, come to believe that it was an anxiety-provoking situation. In this way her anxiety could generalize to every situation. Identifying the sources of anxiety would bind it to those sources. The author repeated this idea about the generalization and binding of anxiety until Mrs. G. appeared convinced of its validity.

Then, instead of making a list of stressful situations, the author took out a pad of drawing paper and drew a picture of a woman in the center to represent Mrs. G. Then he drew pictures of her ex-husband, her daughter, her employer, her automobile, and other people and situations in her life. They were labelled and depicted in such ways that they graphically expressed conflicts and tensions in her life. For example, her husband was depicted as yelling in Mrs. G.'s ear and hitting her; meanwhile she held onto her daughter, who kicked her in the legs, while Mrs. G.'s mother pulled on the child's other hand. Also depicted were problems with her boss, her automobile, her weight, and so on. Balloons were also drawn over the heads of the characters in the depiction which contained pertinent dialogue.

Once the picture was complete, the author reviewed it with her, pointing out each of the binds, problems, and stresses impinging on her. He repeated the suggestion that she now knew that these were the sources of her anxiety and no longer needed to assume that other situations caused the anxiety. He went on to suggest that now that these stressful situations were on paper in the form of a picture, and now that she knew exactly what they were, she might find, as many others had, that the picture could contain the anxiety, including any needless worrying about the problems. That is, she could leave the problems on paper and not take them with her. The therapist then told her that she could take this picture with her, to be used whenever she wished, to help her decide what problems she wished to address and when; and that this would allow her to feel less anxious at those times when her attention was not focused on the picture.

Thus far the effective ingredients of the intervention were believed to consist of the following: 1) the suggestion that identification of the sources of anxiety would bind anxiety; 2) actual binding of anxiety to the degree that there is validity in this notion; 3) containing or binding anxiety by suggesting a transformation of the context in which the anxiety was experienced, i.e., to that of the picture; 4) use of drawing in a ritualistic fashion to accentuate the suggestion that this process of anxiety-binding would produce a positive therapeutic effect; and 5) identifying or naming the problem, by limiting it to those sources of anxiety which were identified.

The practice of giving a name or diagnosis to a problem is sometimes an effective method for producing some relief about problems, especially when the sufferer is uncertain about what is wrong, ruminates about it, and fears the worst. Having a name for the problem sometimes enables the sufferer to more calmly endure the suffering and fosters the belief that the healer knows what to do to help alleviate the problem. It is a method that has been practiced with great skill by shamans and "witch-doctors" in a variety of cultures (Torrey, 1972). It is also commonly practiced in Western cultures, sometimes intentionally and with skill, by physicians and mental health professionals.

The visual illustration of problems by means of cartooning and drawing is usually discussed in the literature in regard to the client being the one to do drawings, not the therapist. However, the author has found a variety of clinical uses for therapist-drawings. While each of these uses take on a different format and have special purposes, in all such uses visual illustration serves to make rapid and resonant linkages to a person's associational system; this avoids the need to communicate by means of a sequence of discrete verbal units in a linear form which may not be processed in the ways intended by the therapist.

Following this first stage of the intervention, the author initiated a second stage during the session by reminding Mrs. G. that she had been feeling a need to handle stress with less anxiety on a more general basis;

and that this constituted a goal for a fundamental change in her life. He then delivered a monologue containing a series of suggestions. He suggested that Mrs. G. might be sensing that a fundamental change was even now occurring or was about to occur, not in just one problem or two, but in her general manner of functioning.

He remarked that this change might be due to fatigue from struggling with each problem over the years as if it were a life or death issue and due also to the realization that each problem was in fact not so very momentous. After all, she could look back on past problems and see now that they were not as catastrophic as she had anticipated. It was suggested that she could see now that perhaps she did not need to look forward anymore to addressing each new stress as if it were a life or death struggle, unless for some reason she needed to continue struggling in this way and needed to feel overwhelmed with the possibility of losing each struggle. If not, then perhaps she was sensing a readiness to give up such struggles and instead focus her attention on allowing herself to discover what the nature of this change was that was about to occur or even was already beginning to occur.

It was stressed that fundamental changes of this kind did not depend on conscious effort and struggle. Conscious effort could be used instead to try to notice the nature of the change. Struggle might be important in other respects, but was unnecessary here; when this change occurred, it would feel to her as if it was happening on its own. It was suggested that she would begin, more and more, to see things differently; and that she would feel more calm, and approach each problem or each stress with a more useful and accurate view of herself and of the world, seeing that each problem was not a life or death issue; and that what she did about it and her role in it, while important, was not all-important. She would not need to struggle to see things in this way and could allow the change to occur in its own time and in its own way.

These suggestions ended the session. They were very similar to the suggestions made to Mr. A. in the previous case example, suggestions which were intended to catalyze a change in self concept regarding vocational competence. Here it was suggested that Mrs. G.'s way of viewing stresses would alter so that she would become less anxious about them. The nature of this change in viewing stress was also specified, utilizing a cognitive restructuring approach (e.g., Ellis, 1977). In this approach, irrational logic and unrealistic expectations are disputed and replaced by more rational ideas. However, these ideas were not applied in a manner typical of cognitive restructuring therapies. Rather than disputing Mrs.

G.'s irrational catastrophizing, the author gave her credit for "sensing" the development of more rational thoughts, which were then described to her.

In both this case and the case of Mr. A. in the previous case example, the suggestion was given that the attitudinal change would occur so subtly that it would be difficult to notice and that it would not occur as a result of conscious efforts to bring it about. This preserved the author from being discredited if the attitudinal change did not occur. It also probably reduced the anxiety which is sometimes occasioned by the client feeling pressured to make an important change happen; it was also intended to instill hope and establish an expectation and attentional set for such a change. The expectation and attentional set were intended to shape, reinforce, and validate any movements in the desired direction, even accidental or random movement.

In this case, one of the reasons that the author gave suggestions for attitudinal change was that he was not yet sure what else he would do to attempt to help Mrs. G. He hoped that he could plant this seed for change and provide a context in which he could, at the least, facilitate a placebo effect. Although it was hoped that the anxiety-binding ritual, as well as other methods the author might use in future sessions, would help to reduce anxiety, the author did not feel he could count on these measures in this case. It was also uncertain whether the ritual would be successful in establishing a clear focus for future treatment, as was intended.

In the next session, Mrs. G. reported that she had experienced a better week and felt less anxious. However, while some improvement occurred in sustaining a focus on particular problems, Mrs. G. still displayed a strong tendency to shift from problem to problem. In subsequent sessions, the author pursued a variety of approaches and tactics but always remained unclear about which aspect of his behavior, advice, or methods were effective. Mrs. G. often benefited in some way from remarks the author had not intended as having major therapeutic value and sometimes she clearly did not benefit from specific attempts by the author to help her with certain problems. Yet, over the course of four months, she gradually improved. The various problems in her life were resolved, either through her own efforts or by accident, and her level of anxiety appeared to fall within a normal range for the first time in over five years. In regard to her style of functioning, she reported that she no longer felt like a "scatterbrain."

Throughout the course of therapy, and even after Mrs. G. terminated, the author continued to review his therapy notes in an effort to determine to his satisfaction what the effective ingredients had been in the therapy that would best account for Mrs. G.'s improvement. The anxiety-binding ritual and the suggestions for attitudinal change which were used in the second session had almost been forgotten by the author and were among a number of other likely possibilities. It is possible that they did play an important role, but this remains uncertain.

Uncertainty of this kind exists in all cases, since therapists can never be sure of the effective ingredients in their therapy. The degree of uncertainty varies from case to case. The author's uncertainty in this case is typical of more cases than one would suppose if judging only from the cases illustrated in the literature. Frequently, therapists put forth their best efforts and use good technique, remain quite uncertain as to whether their interventions are taking hold, and yet observe improvements which are difficult to explain. It is a humbling experience but a typical one. The case of Mrs. G. was included for presentation here for these reasons.

It is possible in cases such as this that improvement occurs as a result either of the placebo effect, or of the beneficial aspects of a therapeutic relationship, or of specific therapist skills and techniques, or of some combination of the above. This uncertainty does not imply that specific techniques are wasted and are not worth further refinement; after all, it is possible that the hypnotic methods used in the case of Mrs. G. were the most effective ingredients. It does imply that the therapist should take some care to establish the kind of therapeutic relationship which by itself can facilitate some improvement, that which was described in Chapter Four and which has also been described in diverse terminology by others (e.g., Bordin, 1979; Hutt, 1976; Hynan, 1981). It also implies that the therapist not interfere with, and even help to create, conditions which might facilitate a placebo effect. Finally, when this kind of therapeutic context has been established, it is more probable, though far from certain, that specific techniques will take hold.

Case 10: Altering Angry Arguments

This case example illustrates the use of storytelling for the purpose of altering people's views of one another, views which engender anger and conflict. The story used here provides an imagery technique which can be considered a form of cognitive restructuring. This particular story has been used in numerous cases where problems concerned control of temper in the escalation of conflict between people. Sometimes the therapeutic sessions involved whole families, sometimes conflictual couples, sometimes a conflictual parent and child, and sometimes an individual who wished to alter his or her conflictual interactions with someone not present.

In all of these cases, other interventions had already been applied to address the problem of anger development and the escalation of conflict. Previous interventions sometimes included the behavioral method of systematic desensitization, psychodynamic methods which addressed sources of unrealistic rage, and family therapy methods aimed at the context which maintained the conflicts. Interventions also included strategies developed by the MRI group (Fisch et al., 1982) for problems they described as "reaching accord through opposition" and "confirming the accuser's suspicions by defending oneself"; these usually consisted of providing a rationale for one or the other party to take a one-down position and thereby interrupt a predictable sequence of escalating conflict consisting of one-upmanship maneuvers on both sides.

Other interventions included the teaching of Ginott's (1969) rules for constructive expression of anger and some "psychotechniques" compiled by Didato (1981). Also used was Gordon's approach (1976) of teaching "I-messages" for expressing the hurt feelings that lead to defensive anger, imagery techniques developed by Lazarus (1977), and the cognitive restructuring techniques developed by Ellis (1977) to alter a person's expectations of others.

Although all of these techniques are useful in a great many cases, there are some cases in which they seem to have little effect despite clients' best efforts to understand and to learn them. One reason some clients find these methods so difficult to apply is that they require the learning of complicated sequences of cognitions, learning which is often too recent and too fragile for use in the face of an anger-provoking situation and which is not well enough rehearsed or internalized to be easily accessed in the heat of battle. Clients often find that the battle is already upon them before they realize that it is an appropriate occasion to apply the new learning. By that time it is often too late to successfully apply the new learning because their intense feelings and overlearned interactional habits have caught them up in circular sequences of escalating conflict.

For example, one woman was able to learn in the therapy sessions that it was quite demanding to expect life to be fair to her and to expect that her husband should know better than to flirt with other women. These expectations and beliefs tended to work her into a rage. She was taught to say to herself, repeatedly, that life was not fair, and that unpleasant events were expected, and that her husband could be expected to behave in displeasing ways due to his ignorance and due to his emotional disturbance. This is a somewhat simplistic example of cognitive restructuring methods but it illustrates the point that a client could be taught to alter her expectations by practicing self talk that was unusual for her. Yet, even after she practiced at home, the complicated differences between the new and the old self talk were such that the new learning was insufficiently internalized and not readily accessible in the midst of an intense provocation. Even when she began the new train of thinking, there were too many points where it broke down before it could result in altered expectations.

This can be viewed as a technical problem in the refinement of therapeutic applications of methods. It can be addressed, behaviorally, by increased homework and practice, at the risk of boring clients and driving them from therapy. However, it is sometimes possible to find a way to telescope the complicated cognitions necessary to alter expectations into a single and powerful image. This is accomplished in the story illustrated below.

In the case used for illustration, the main conflict existed between father and son, and it was so intense that it escalated to near-violence at times. However, this conflict detoured the mother's conflict with the father, masking the spousal conflict when it became too intense. The father-son conflict was used mainly by the mother for this reason, but was used by the father too in reaction to the father's jealousy of the mother's alliance with and support of the son. Occasionally, intense conflict erupted between mother and son, recapitulating the father-mother conflict because the son was viewed by the mother as a replica of the father.

Therefore, the story was directed at all three of them, hoping it might affect each to varying extents. The story was not the only intervention used; its use was based on the failure of various interventions to take hold which were described above, some of which consisted of cognitive restructuring methods aimed at altering expectations. It should be pointed out that the mother and son often accused the father of being "crazy" and needing "deep" therapy, and that the father often accused the son of being "crazy" as well. These accusations were justified in their minds by the demonstrations of explosive anger each had witnessed in the past.

The author pointed out to the family in this session that many techniques had been attempted to help each of them to alter their expectations of the other and that these had all had some effect but had basically failed to prevent an escalation of angry conflict. He said that this failure might be due to the difficulty in carrying out the complicated sequence of thoughts that would make the techniques work and that only very diligent rehearsal and homework would succeed. He said that he was unsure the family was willing to put that degree of effort into changing and if they weren't, then they as well as the author ought to just give up trying to make these particular techniques work. He then pointed out that this situation reminded him of a story he remembered of a problem that a friend of his had a long, long time ago.

The above comments conveyed a message of impotence; that is, that perhaps the author could not help the clients to change with the techniques he had thus far offered because the way they had attempted to apply the techniques had clearly been unsuccessful. This is equivalent to the message of "Don't try to change in this way any longer." Yet, the message that change will occur is implicitly conveyed by the fact that the author continues to sit in the session to tell a story as if this will somehow help the clients. Also, it is a story intended to provide further opportunity for change to occur and this expectation was probably communicated in tone and attitude. The announcement of a story highlights the message that they should give up conscious efforts to master complicated techniques, and instead simply relax and listen. A story about something that happened "a long time ago" also redistributes attention, distracting attention from current concerns.

The author then told the family about a friend, who was, at the time of the story, a young psychologist who had just spent five years in graduate school. The story is paraphrased below.

My friend had just finished studying many interesting and effective psychological techniques in graduate school. He had spent four years of undergraduate school and then five years of graduate work in learning about how people think and feel and learn and remember and change. However, he hadn't practiced the knowledge and techniques he had learned, except on himself, and he wasn't very experienced. As part of his graduate program, he had to do an internship in which he would get the opportunity to begin to apply the things he had learned. His internship was in a hospital and he enjoyed the experience very much because finally he was able to practice some of the things he'd studied so hard to learn. He was always studying new psychological techniques and would practice them on himself in order to improve himself in a variety of ways. As a result, he was usually kind, patient, understanding, and never got very angry because he was very good at understanding the sources of his anger and dealing with these sources in appropriate psychological ways.

Except when he visited his mother-in-law. Whenever he visited his mother-in-law, he would always end up acting like a raving maniac. Here was a young man who hardly ever got angry and all he had to do is see his mother-in-law to become screaming mad.

At this point in the story, the father laughed, saying, "That will do it every time." Then he and his wife exchanged a joke about their in-laws. The author then went on with the story.

Whenever this young psychologist visited this woman, he ended up yelling, screaming, ranting, and raving. He would do his best to remain calm and try to stay out of arguments, but each time, she would say or do something that would absolutely infuriate him and he would lose all self control and begin arguing with her, and before he knew it, he was firing off strings of curses like a maniac. He was horribly ashamed of himself. Here he was, a young psychologist who had all these sophisticated psychological techniques available to him to deal with anger who was behaving in what he considered to be a most shameful manner. He liked to think of himself as the kind of person who could practice what he preached.

And so he tried using all those psychological methods. He would practice at home all the time, where he would visualize his mother-in-law while he rehearsed many things to himself about how he could not expect her to behave the way he wished her to behave and many other useful trains of thought derived from cognitive restructuring and imagery approaches. He would get so he felt quite confident he could handle her when he saw her again. Then he'd go over there to visit and when she said or did something that infuriated him, he would start using his methods. For example, one method he tried was identical to one that you all tried. He would try to lower his expectations of his mother-in-law by saying to himself, "Who says she's got to behave the way I want her to? How can she? Lots of people, like her, are ignorant and stupid and disturbed and that's how they behave. It would be nice if she were different, but it's not awful if she's not the way I wish and there's no universal law that says she should be." Does it sound familiar?

Whenever this young man found himself getting mad at his mother-in-law, he tried using this sort of method to help lower his expectations, but it would take too long, and he could only listen to himself with one ear and couldn't quite get it right because he'd get so involved in the situation that he'd just forget all of these psychological techniques and become a raving maniac once again. All his efforts to solve the problem were failing, so he finally figured he'd have to give up trying. And he did give up and accepted the fact that he was just a miserable worm like the rest of us who was fated to commit shameful acts towards others from time to time.

And then one day at the hospital he was talking to a disturbed patient who was saying some pretty nasty things to him, and suddenly he realized something surprising and yet not so very surprising after all. He realized that he never got angry at these patients, even though they said some things that were just as provocative as his mother-in-law said to him, and he realized why. It was because they were patients and he didn't take what they said personally. They were disturbed, and therefore they were expected to behave in this way. He did not have to go through a complicated sequence of thoughts to realize this every time he talked to a patient. He just knew all these things every time he looked at a patient. The problem was that he didn't just automatically know all these things when he looked at his mother-in-law.

Instead, he was viewing and treating his mother-in-law like a normal person, expecting her to behave like a normal person, the way he expected normal people to behave, expecting her to behave as he wished her to behave rather than the way she really behaved. And he considered that the way she really behaved was just as disturbed as his patients and he knew that he could expect her to behave in these ways rather than the ways he wished she would behave. He had known this all along and had tried telling himself this with his psychological techniques of self-talk but it hadn't worked because she was so good at conveying the image of a normal, decent, rational human being, at least what he considered normal. Actually, she was an artist at getting him to believe she was what he considered normal. And this would fool him into believing it every time, so that when she then behaved like a disturbed person, he would react by thinking that she shouldn't behave that way and that she should know better and should be punished for behaving in such ways, which was his way of working himself into a righteous rage.

What he needed to do was treat her like a patient, and he needed a quick and easy way to remember to treat her as a patient, just as he unconsciously and automatically lowered his expectations of his patients. He didn't need a lot of sophisticated psychological self talk. So he tried picturing an image in his mind of his mother-in-law as a patient wearing a hospital gown, and he laughed at how easy it was to imagine her as a mental patient in that hospital gown. After all, he had always thought she was crazy anyway, even though he figured she was an artist at getting him to treat her as normal. He imagined her in that hospital gown, walking around her house and doing chores and cooking and cleaning and talking to the family and still wearing that white gown that showed that she was a patient.

And then, the next time he went to visit, as soon as he laid eyes on his mother-in-law, he pictured that she had that hospital gown under her clothes and had escaped from the psychiatric ward. And by thinking that she might have that hospital gown under her clothes, he ended up thinking, "She's a patient, she's disturbed, don't be fooled by what she does." And an amazing thing happened.

He found himself treating her differently, with gentleness and kindness and tolerance. And even when she tried goading him into arguments, it just didn't work anymore because he figured that the gown was there under her clothes, which reminded him of how disturbed she was. And he didn't need alot of techniques because that one image in his head changed all his expectations of his mother-in-law in an instant, better than all the other psychological techniques put together. He just needed that one image in his head. That's all.

Throughout the rendition of this story, the family members appeared extremely attentive and when the story was over they were quiet and thoughtful. An appointment was made almost immediately afterwards, without any substantive discussion of anything else. This allowed the story to work on them without interference from analysis and discussion. The scheduling of another appointment also helped to maintain the message that change would occur.

In subsequent sessions, comments were sometimes made by the mother and son about the story which indicated that each had made use of it in their own different ways, and that it had helped at times to alter their views enough to alter an escalation of anger. This was enough at times to interrupt or prevent conflictual sequences of interaction with the father, who appeared to be entirely unaffected by the story.

This story is used in different ways in different cases, sometimes being told with elaborate detail to fulfill certain other hypnotic and therapeutic functions. Sometimes it has had no apparent effects, but other times it has seemed to have a useful effect. It is hoped that stories of this kind, containing images which contract or truncate the effective ingredients of cognitive restructuring techniques, may be useful to other therapists. I also hope that the hypnotic functions that are fulfilled in interventions of this kind were made evident in this illustration.

Case 11: Altering a Relationship with Food (with a transcript of an audio cassette)

Ms. V. was a thirty six year old single parent when she called the author for help in losing weight and with complaints of depression, job dissatisfaction, and lack of motivation for doing anything to address her problems. She said that she also wanted help for her adolescent daughter's weight problem, but that her daughter refused to come in. Since Ms. V.

was so unmotivated to do anything about her problems, calling the author had been a big step forward in her view and she doubted that she would be taking any other big steps too quickly. She did not think she was motivated enough to begin a diet and she hoped that she might develop sufficient motivation in therapy.

The first session consisted mainly of assessment of the various problems. It became apparent that Ms. V. had been on diets most of her life, losing and gaining a great deal of weight over and over again throughout the years. She had used diet pills, had been involved in numerous weight control programs, and had used a number of distinct diet plans. Most of these measures were initially effective but Ms. V. would always relapse and gain back every pound she had lost. She had been steadily gaining weight for the past several years, ever since she began work in an office of the state department of mental health. She hated her work and claimed that most of her co-workers also hated their work, but that they were all trapped in their jobs by the good pay and benefits. She described the work setting as "adult day care" because very little work got done and most of each day was spent socializing and creating a pretense of work.

Unlike many other individuals treated by the author for eating problems, Ms. V. did not overeat at home. She overate at work, where she and her co-workers ate at a fairly steady pace throughout the workday. According to her description, two thirds of the staff were overweight in her office and offices associated with hers in the department of mental health. In her own office there was a refrigerator, a microwave oven, a toaster, a popcorn popper, an array of condiments, pots, pans, eating utensils and napkins. She described one man's desk as a pantry and another's as a miniature grocery store. The office was stocked with supplies of soda, juice, hot dogs, and other foods too numerous to itemize.

She and her co-workers did not simply snack on doughnuts in the morning as is done in many offices. They enjoyed many meals each day, as well as snacks. These included quiches, sandwiches, pasta, hot dogs, pizza, ice cream, salads, cookies, fudge, juices, candy, and anything else they had a taste for. In addition, Ms. V. usually went out for a big lunch with some of her co-workers, following which they would stop at a bakery or a fudge shop for dessert. Aside from eating three meals a day, she was probably eating the equivalent of four or five meals during working hours.

Aside from other interventions which addressed her depression and her vocational dissatisfaction, the author addressed Ms. V.'s eating problems in the second session. He made sure that she was in good health and that increased exercise and reduced intake of food was sanctioned by her physician. He then explored with her various types of exercise to find those that appealed to her and which she could permanently integrate into her life. He discussed the values of exercise with her, pointing out that it burned calories and increased the metabolic rate throughout the rest of the day so that more calories would be burned even when not exercising. He also pointed out that it increased muscle tone and fitness and provided a psychological sense of well being.

He then provided Ms. V. with some suggestions which were aimed at altering her relationship with food. The suggestions were indirect only in the sense that Ms. V. was told that there was an approach available to her when she was ready to use it but that the author did not know if she was ready yet. He told her a bit about the approach but was careful not to ask her to use it. He even restrained her from using it until she was ready and motivated to do so.

The approach is an integration of methods taken from Milton Erickson, Theodore Barber, behavior approaches to weight reduction, and some of the professional literature on weight control. It consists of a number of components, some of which are more or less relevant for different individuals. Primarily it asks that the person stop struggling with the conflict of whether to eat or not, since this maintains a love-hate relationship with food and defines oneself in terms of eating. The person is asked to give up this struggle and to eat whenever she wishes. However, when she eats, she is to eat in a different way than usual.

Instead of dumping food into her body while attention is placed on something else, she is to place full attention on the process of eating and is to eat slowly, savoring each bite and extracting all the pleasure from the process. In this way a positive relationship towards food and eating can be established, rather than one associated with either overindulgence or deprivation. It is suggested further that if food is eaten in this way, the person will find that she will not really eat much at all because she will notice she has had enough and will also discover she does not really like the taste of certain foods that she thought she had liked.

Rapid weight loss would be a sign that the person was not following the approach properly and was trying too hard and probably depriving herself, and thereby maintaining a struggle with food. It is emphasized that this is an approach that can be permanently integrated into one's life so that food can be enjoyed and thought about and so that one can gradually achieve an ideal weight and stay at it, without a painful struggle. Sometimes it is important to address childhood conditioning, in which

a person learned to eat as an expression of defiance and control. Sometimes, eating meets other needs, and these are addressed by helping the
client to discover more appropriate ways to meet those needs.

In the case of Ms. V., this approach was described in rather sketchy
terms in the second session. When she returned to the third session, she
had begun a daily exercise program and had acted on the suggestion about
eating. She had stopped eating at work, and as a result, her caloric intake
had been dramatically reduced. She did not feel deprived because she
knew she could eat whenever she liked and had experimented with eating
in this permissive way. She had tried eating during work hours, but doing
so slowly and with full attention on the eating had resulted in her putting
the food down. The author pointed out that she was in the perfect work
setting for implementing and mastering this approach because she would
not be able to avoid food. The constant presence of food and the negative
examples of co-workers who constantly went off their many types of diet
would provide an excellent context for learning the new approach.

Subsequent sessions were spent monitoring her progress, and reinforcing and highlighting various aspects of the approach. For example,
she was doing so well that at one point the author suggested a relapse
(that is, to dump food into her body without placing attention on the
process of eating), so that she could vividly recall her previous approach
to food and compare it to her present approach. This also demonstrated
that eating less is not an all or nothing affair; that relapses were expected
and did not put an end to the approach.

She also remained fearful of a binge, so the author suggested she go
ahead and have one whenever the impulse hit her. He suggested that she
would find it difficult to complete the binge in the same way as she used
to, because she was developing habits of fully attending to the process
of eating, and would discover interesting things the next time she binged.
When she next began to binge, sitting down late one night with a box
of chocolate chip cookies and a half gallon of ice cream, she discovered
after a couple of cookies and a few spoonfuls of ice cream that she had
extracted all the taste she wanted and didn't really feel like eating any
further.

She found herself forgetting the approach and lapsing back to dumping
food in her body whenever she ate with someone else. The author pointed
out that this was natural, since conversation and social interaction necessarily distracts attention from the process of eating and tasting. The
author also pointed out that this was an unfortunate and wasteful situation
because all those calories were getting dumped in her body and she wasn't

even getting the benefit of enjoying them. He provided two suggestions to resolve the dilemma. First, she could try to develop the habit of putting her fork down while talking. If this proved to be too difficult to learn or if it did not help, he suggested the more drastic strategy of having only low caloried and tasteless foods when eating socially, since this food would only get dumped into her body anyway. She was to reserve high caloried foods for occasions when she could devote her full attention to enjoying them.

She also found it difficult to make transitions from completing one activity to beginning another, since she had used to eat during transitional moments or when feeling bored. The author suggested experimenting with consumption of liquid, preferably spring water, and with perhaps a dash of lemon juice. This quickly became a habit for her.

Genuine relapses, in which she ate without thinking, were rare, but when they occurred she experienced guilt, despite the author's best efforts to encourage a guilt-free approach to eating. The guilt was a carry-over from previous dieting approaches in which it played a role in perpetuating a diet-binge cycle, a cycle which can be described in the following way. The responsible adult in her would eat appropriately for awhile until the defiant and impulsive child in her had had quite enough deprivation and would take over on a binge. The binge would be followed by an over-whelming sense of guilt where the adult again took over and deprived the child.

The author worried that the presence of guilt was an anchor to her previous approach and could catalyze a resumption of it at some point if it was not neutralized. Therefore he told her that if she insisted on punishing herself with feeling guilty, then she could do it overtly by engaging in a boring exercise for the time it took to burn off the calories she had consumed. For example, if she had eaten a bagel (about 150 calories) while her attention was on something other than enjoying the bagel, she could punish herself by briskly walking up and down a hallway for 30 minutes (since brisk walking burns about five calories per minute). This would assuage her guilt, rather than the guilt being left to tempt her to deprive herself. It would also be good for her body. A boring exercise was stipulated rather than one she enjoyed so that it would be punishing and so that the exercises she was permanently integrating in her life would not become associated with punishment. She attempted this task a few times and finally gave it up, finding it to be a silly ordeal. However, it also helped her to give up her guilt for her rare relapses.

At her request, the author provided her with an audio cassette tape containing the basic suggestions for the approach used. She wanted this for help in reinforcing the approach and also for the purpose of leaving it around the house for her daughter to find and to use. An almost identical monologue is provided on Side 2 of the cassette tape which accompanies this book. A transcript of it appears below. The basic approach reflected in this transcript has been useful to a number of clients who tend to find the struggle-free aspect of it quite different from previous approaches they have tried. Different features are emphasized or underemphasized in each case, depending on the features of the unique situation. Hopefully it will be useful to other therapists who may wish to adapt it in their own ways to eating problems.

Transcript

I'd like to describe a way of thinking about living and about eating that you can find helpful in achieving your goals but you can find your own ways to make the best use of these thoughts. And you can begin to put these thoughts into practice whenever you fully understand that you have all the resources you need for this to work for you. And whenever you really understand that you don't have to use will power or grit your teeth or deprive yourself of all the things you want to eat. You've already struggled long enough with food in this way.

In fact, your struggle with food can be described as a conflict, a relationship of conflict between food and yourself. You've always found yourself in the conflict of deciding whether to give into temptation or not to give in, to eat or not to eat. By putting yourself into a conflict with food, you end up always defining yourself as either a person who has just resisted the temptation or as a person who has just given in to the temptation. Do you want to go on forever defining yourself in terms of eating? In terms of whether you're fat or thin? In terms of dieting or giving in to temptation? Do you want to give food that kind of power over you?

This struggle with food, this conflictual relationship with food, is a love-hate relationship that I think is very painful for you. I would be doing you an injustice if I asked you to continue the struggle by telling you to go on another diet like you have in the past. Each diet that you've been on may have been this kind of a struggle where it seemed like you were winning for a time, but then you'd give in and end up feeling like a failure. You've gained pounds and lost pounds and gained them and lost them back again and you know how frustrating and unhealthy this can be. But you probably never realized that there's a way that you can give up this painful struggle with food, a way that's available to you because it requires skills and knowledge you already have. You'll soon understand that you can give up all that struggling and that you can establish a different relationship to food. A positive relationship of love and respect.

The first thing to realize is that wanting to eat or not wanting to eat is not within your voluntary control. Think about that and you'll see that it's so. You can't just make yourself not want to eat by an act of will power. That's what you've tried doing in the past. And what happens is that your will power breaks down at some point, and before you know it you find yourself unthinkingly dumping food into your body. And you do just dump food into your body, because usually you're paying attention to something else, and not paying full attention to the food and to the process of eating.

Rather than eating because you're hungry and for the purpose of enjoying eating and getting all the taste out of it, maybe you're doing it for some other reason. Perhaps because you're bored, perhaps because you feel you need to give something nice to yourself, maybe because you feel deprived, or feel a sense of emptiness, maybe to feel more solid and secure, maybe to express a sense of defiance at being pushed around and controlled by others. Whatever the reason is, you keep on dumping food in your body. And you may think you're enjoying it. But do you really think you're enjoying it all you can? My guess is that your attention isn't completely focused on the process of eating and that you may be eating too fast to fully enjoy it. When your attention is on other things and when you eat too fast, then what you're doing is just dumping lots of calories into your body and misusing yourself, and missing out on all of the enjoyment you could have gotten out of the experience of eating.

I think you can begin to see what I'm getting at. You may not be able to control whether you want to eat, but you can control how you eat, whether you eat slowly or quickly and whether you place your attention on eating or on something else, like reading or T.V. or a conversation. So if you want to give up this love-hate relationship with food in which you go on struggling with it all the time, then you've got to understand, really understand, that you can feel free to eat. You don't have to try not to eat. You can't accomplish your purpose that way. Instead you can just feel free to go ahead and eat whenever you want to. But when you do eat, you can do it differently than before. Do you realize that if you eat slowly and if you place your full attention on the eating then you'll get all the enjoyment out of it that's there and that in the process you'll end up losing weight? This is something within your voluntary control. Eating slowly and with full attention on eating.

And when you eat in this way, do you realize you can discover new things. For one thing, you can discover that you don't want to eat as much food as you used to. You simply don't need to because you'll be getting all the taste and satisfaction that's there. And when you discover this you can take pleasure in the fact that it's so easy to eat and to live in this way. And you can also discover new tastes that you find you like and also find, now that you're really tasting the food, that you don't really like the taste of certain foods as much as you thought you did. And you can develop a habit of eating in this way, slowly and with full attention on it. And once it becomes a habit, you'll find that you don't have to struggle any longer with whether to eat or not, and you won't have to keep losing and gaining and losing and gaining. This is a permanent approach towards living and eating. It's the establishment of a positive relationship with food, to replace your conflictual relationship of struggling with whether to eat or not to eat. And little by little, not rapidly, you can achieve an ideal body size, without a struggle. Think of what it will be like and how you'll look at an ideal body size.

I hope you understand that the process of losing weight and living at an ideal body size is not just trying to eat less. It's a process of learning to think and to live in a different way. To think differently about ourselves and about eating and to establish a better relationship to food, not to deprive ourselves of it. When we eat, we can concentrate on eating and thoroughly enjoy it, slowly, undistracted by other things, and we can get all of the satisfaction out of the food that's in there. Do you know that if you concentrate enough just on eating, that time may even seem to slow down so that the simple process of eating a sandwich can seem like a full course dinner, if you eat slowly and with deliberation and concentration on the enjoyment of each bite. You probably didn't realize that you could lose weight in such an enjoyable way.

Do you know how enjoyable it is to eat in this way? Not to just shovel the food down as fast as you can. There's no need to hurry. You can string out the pleasure. When you eat in this way you treat your body with respect, respect for your body's capacities to give you the pleasure of tastes and respect for its capacities to convert that food to energy. Your tongue is there with its hundreds of taste buds to enable you to appreciate all the different kinds of tastes there are and to fully enjoy the food. And your body contains all the teeth and chemicals and enzymes it needs to break down the food and convert it to energy. And the food itself is worthy of respect for the complicated way in which it's put together to provide us with proteins, vitamins, energy, and all the sustenance that we need. You can treat it with respect and can savor each bit of it, enjoy the sight of it, the feel of it in your mouth. You can eat like a gourmet, even when eating an ordinary sandwich. Each time you eat is an opportunity to meditate on the remarkable capacities of your body and on the complicated nature of food itself. Each act of eating is an opportunity to meditate on these things. I don't have to give you any self hypnosis ritual to remind you of these things. Each act of eating can be a reminder as you learn to treat food and your body in this more respectful way.

As you find in yourself ways to use this approach, please don't do so with any kind of rigid diet. You've been on many diets and you probably know all about how many calories are in each food and what meal plan constitutes a well balanced and nutritious diet. You've become an expert at it and you can use this expertise to plan your meals and to enjoy thinking about and planning to eat different foods. You can think of all the different foods with low caloric value and plan which ones you wish to eat and which ones your body enjoys. You know best what you like and what's good for you. And you can think of high caloried foods as well, and plan how to integrate them into your day and plan on really extracting all the pleasure from them in order to make it really worth those calories. Planning can be useful because it helps to make for a well balanced diet and it helps to remind you not to unthinkingly dump lots of calories into your body without fully enjoying the food. And planning and thinking about what to eat is fun. It's the opposite of trying not to think about food. You can think about it all you like. But don't overplan either. You'll know you're overplanning if you even begin to feel that you're depriving yourself. You don't have to deprive yourself. You only have to fully appreciate food and realize the enjoyment in eating. Do you see now how this can be fun? That it can be a strictly positive experience with no pain and deprivation.

In learning to live differently and to think differently about yourself and your life and about eating, you probably already know that it helps to regularly engage in exercise and activity. Nothing excessive that will cause aches and pains because that also is an abuse of our bodies, an abuse of a body that is helpless and dependent on our good judgement about how we care for it, how we feed it, how we rest it, and how we exercise it. Taking your body for a walk or a healthy workout can help you to become aware of all the muscles and organs and miraculous workings of your body, and to treat it with more respect and tenderness, and to realize you can achieve an ideal body size that you can permanently enjoy.

As you carry out this approach you may realize more clearly the reasons why you used to eat and that you mislabeled other needs and feelings for a need to eat. A need for companionship or love. A need to defy someone. A need to fill emptiness or boredom. Every time you have a need to eat, you can notice whether there are other needs that can be addressed and perhaps you can begin to take measures to address the needs, rather than misusing and abusing your body to address them by unthinkingly dumping food into it.

You don't need to try to remember all of these things to carry out this approach. You may find yourself interested in one aspect of it on one day, and another aspect of it on another day, and develop your own ways to understand and to add to the approach. You only need to remember to eat slowly and with full attention on enjoyment of the food. You may even forget these simple instructions because they are so contrary to all the habits you've developed and contrary to other diet advice you've heard in the past. But each time you do remember to eat in this way, even if it's only once in awhile, you'll be engaging in the process of developing these new habits, habits that can become a permanent approach to eating and to living. And once these are habits, you can rest on them and just coast, fully enjoying this relationship to food. You'll have established a relationship to food that is entirely a positive, loving, reverent relationship, reflecting a respect for food and a respect for yourself, and you can leave behind you that painful struggle of whether to eat or not to eat. Do you realize that you can even enjoy this relationship right now if you like? Have something to eat and see.

Discussion

Although various hypnotic methods and principles were applied in each case, the relative prominence of each principle varied from case to case. For example, pacing and leading were processes illustrated in the case of *The Chores of Life,* but the intervention in that case depended most on redistribution of attention. In contrast, the intervention applied in the case of *Mental Retardation* depended heavily on pacing and leading. Distraction was also prominent in *Mental Retardation* and it is interesting that its function can be subsumed within the concept of redistribution of attention, which was prominent in *Chores.* Yet, the application of this broad concept was quite different in the two cases: in *Mental Retardation* the function was that of distraction from leading maneuvers, whereas in *Chores* the function was that of altering the subjective perception of an experience.

The perception of behavior and change occurring on its own or involuntarily was suggested in most of the cases, either verbally or implicitly. This message was communicated most prominently and emphatically in those cases involving ritual, most notably the cases of *Impotence* and *Generalized Anxiety Disorder.* In *Impotence,* a ritualistic game was prescribed; in *Anxiety,* the anxiety-binding procedure of drawing was utilized as a ritual. When ritual is used, a clear but implicit nonverbal message is conveyed that performance of the ritual will result in the desired change. Explicit verbal suggestions to this effect serve only to clarify and augment the implicit suggestions conveyed by ritual.

In most cases, especially the last one on *Altering a Relationship to Food,* it was evident that a person's relationship to a problem could be understood as a symmetrical struggle with that problem. Therapeutic comments and suggestions which punctuate the notion that continued struggle is useless can help a person to give up that struggle and to place attention and energy in more constructive directions. Continued struggle can interfere with both the therapist's and the client's attempts to bring about significant therapeutic change. Giving up the struggle also helps to alter the person's relationship to the problem, from a symmetrical to a complementary relationship. This change dovetails with therapist suggestions, either explicit or implicit, to allow the change to feel as if it is occurring effortlessly and on its own.

To successfully make such suggestions, the therapist must avoid engagement in either a complementary or a symmetrical relationship with the client. To avoid this, it is necessary for the therapist to interact with the client in such a way that the client does not have to make conscious or deliberate attempts to get rid of the problem, for example, to lose weight or feel less anxious by an act of will. Attempts of this kind can be considered to be obedient, complementary responses by the client, responses which are not usually possible to make and which would only result in continued struggle with the problem.

If the client should make conscious attempts to behave in this way, for example, by attempting obediently to feel less anxious in response to the therapist's implicit suggestion to feel less anxious, the therapist can tell the client to stop trying to do this. This prevents the relationship from becoming a complementary one. At the same time, if the client engages in a symmetrical maneuver, for example, by complaining that he still feels terribly anxious despite therapeutic suggestions, the therapist must avoid responding in like-fashion with symmetrical maneuvers on his part, for example, by trying to convince the client to feel less anxious. He can instead respond with meta-complementary maneuvers which agree with or pace the client's behaviors.

In this way, the therapist keeps himself from becoming engaged in either a complementary or a symmetrical relationship with the client. When the therapist can in this way remain the one who defines what kind of relationship it is, an optimal interactional context is created for the client to find the capacity to surrender in the symmetrical struggle with the problem and allow change to occur in a manner that feels effortless. Of the cases presented in this chapter, the importance of the therapist maintaining this position is nowhere more clearly illustrated than in the case of *A Therapeutic Mistake* where the author failed to maintain this position.

Concluding Remarks

In looking at this collection of cases, it is interesting to observe that hypnotic methods (as these methods are commonly understood) are more prominent in cases such as *Altering Angry Arguments,* where a story was told to facilitate an alteration in expectations, or *A Problem of Occupational Identity,* where stories were used to suggest attitudinal change. The ways in which hypnotic methods were used in these cases are more clearly recognizable from the hypnosis literature and therefore have the appearance here of being "borrowed" from the field of hypnosis. Yet, hypnotic methods might not be apparent without being pointed out in cases such as *An Obsessive Child, Impotence, Relationship Hopping,* and *Temper Tantrums.* The interventions used in these cases could easily have been explained by other therapy models and without invocation of hypnotic methods.

This comparison between two sets of cases in this collection of cases highlights the question of when one begins, or stops, describing interventions as hypnotic. In some cases, it may be more useful to communicate explanations in more conventional terms and unnecessary to describe the hypnotic aspects. Yet these cases have been included here to illustrate that there is more than a "borrowing" involved when hypnotic methods are being applied. I hope that this collection of cases, in the present chapter as well as previous ones, has made it clear that most therapy is hypnotic and that there is an equivalence between comments made during a family therapy session on who shall have custody of a child and a hypnotic arm levitation.

12

CONCLUSION

While there is some overlap between the purposes of this book and the teaching of an Eriksonian approach to hypnosis, I hope it is evident that a book of this nature cannot possibly do justice to the indirect and subtle approach to hypnosis which is practiced by Ericksonians. Although this sort of subtlety and indirection existed in some of the interventions illustrated, it did not exist in many others where more direct methods were sometimes applied. The subtlety practiced by Erickson can be better learned from those who devote themselves to understanding and applying his particular hypnotic and therapeutic approach. The main purpose of this book has been to demonstrate the application of hypnotic methods, direct as well as indirect, in a variety of therapeutic contexts, even in those which are not ordinarily associated with hypnosis. The book supports, by examples and commentary, the argument advanced by Haley (1963) that most therapy can be considered to be essentially hypnotic in form.

The hypnotic methods illustrated here have included some which are easily recognizable as hypnotic and which result in an appearance of "borrowing" from hypnotherapy. However, they also have included applications which contain only the essence of hypnotic methods; the result has been that these latter applications might not have been recognizable as hypnotic at all without having highlighted what is hypnotic about them. In both types of applications of hypnotic methods, those which were more apparent and those which were less apparent, the irreducible essence of those methods has been described here as the establishment of a particular kind of relationship, with a unique structural form and with a unique sequence of communications between therapist and client. This relationship is evident in any of the case illustrations, in those that are not ordinarily recognizable as hypnotic as well as those containing recognizable hypnotic methods. As was repeatedly noted, when a therapist is able to establish and maintain this kind of relationship, the client is often able to find ways to alter his or her relationship with the problem.

In order to adequately demonstrate the hypnotic nature of most therapies, it was necessary to include applications such as that illustrated in Chapter Eight on child custody mediation because most therapists would not expect hypnotic methods to be usefully applied in cases of spousal conflict, and especially not in the context of a court referred evaluation. Yet it is easy to see the equivalence between the predictable sequence of maneuvers used in that case and those used in the case illustration in Chapter Eleven in which the mentally retarded residents were rapidly maneuvered out of the house. It is also easy to see the equivalence between the sequence of pacing, leading, and distracting maneuvers used in the latter case and those used to produce the nonverbal arm levitation described in Chapter Three.

It is crucial to recognize the equivalence between these interventions because pacing, leading, bi-level messages of change and don't change, and other methods are all maneuvers which might be used in various cases but which might be applied at the wrong moments in an interaction and neglected at those moments when they are necessary. It is not simply the inclusion of these methods in therapy which facilitates change, but rather how these methods are used in an interaction. The interaction must be the kind that locks a client into the direction of change and hotwires reality. Whether subtle forms of pacing and leading are used or whether blunt and direct language is used, the common thread which emerges in all of the case illustrations is the particular pattern of communication and the establishment of a certain form of relationship between the therapist and the system in which the problem is embedded.

In most cases, it is easy to describe the system in which the problem is embedded, whether it consists of an individual with a smoking problem or a problem of impotence in a couple or a spousal conflict. In other cases, it is not so easy. For example, in the case of the mentally retarded residents, I am not sure that either the residents or the staff could be considered to be the "clients" with whom the therapist established a hypnotic relationship. Rather, it was with resident behaviors and features of the situation that this relationship was established to bring about change. A case of this kind challenges our constructs of reality and leads us to question exactly what we mean when we try to define the hypnotic or therapeutic relationship. Its definition here as a paradoxical relationship that is neither symmetrical nor complementary, or as a communication of a bi-level message containing paradoxical injunctions which interface with the client's paradoxical communications, may not be the most apt way to describe it.

After all, once one understands that the message of "Change-don't change" really means "Change but don't change on purpose," the logical paradox or contradiction usually believed to exist in this message is diluted. No longer is "paradox" being used to address "resistance" with rationales involving reverse psychology or control issues. What is conveyed, instead, is an expression of the richness of alternatives and polarities available, which reflects a recognition that right/wrong and other dualities can coexist. Rather than forcing nature into one side of a polarity, for example by attempting to "utilize resistance," the approach can more accurately be understood to capitalize on the coexistence of polarities.

This failure of the concept of paradox to aptly capture the situation is very evident in the mediation case where it is clear that the therapeutic content, or words, used to fulfill the blocking function (i.e., the message "Don't change on purpose") is very unlike the content which fulfills this blocking function in many other therapeutic situations. The message in many other situations is "Don't change on purpose," or "Don't try to get rid of your headache," or "Don't lift your arm with conscious effort." It is equivalent to the blocking function in the mediation case in the sense that the spouses were asked to stop doing what they usually thought to be appropriate to try to accomplish their goals. Yet, what they usually did could hardly be described as "on purpose." They had to use more purpose and effort to bring about the kind of change which has been described as "effortless" in most cases illustrated here.

It is clear that to describe this mediation intervention as a paradoxical "Change-don't change" message is to strain the concept of paradox, much like stretching or mixing metaphors. Yet it is also clear that the repetitive sequences of therapist and client interaction in that intervention are equivalent to hypnotic interactions in other illustrations, such as the arm levitation, in which the concept of paradox more aptly captures what is happening. This is why the approach described here may more accurately be described as a way of capitalizing on polarities. Yet, the terminology and concepts used throughout this book to convey the essential workings of the approach have been deliberately chosen to include concepts such as paradox, contradiction, incongruity, bi-level message, symmetry, complementarity, and so on. The reason for this choice is that this terminology has become conventional in the literature and comprises a language that I can be sure will clearly communicate my essential understandings about therapy and the therapeutic relationship. I don't think that the names we use to describe our understandings matter as much as the understandings themselves.

Although not the most apt, the terminology I have borrowed from Bateson, Haley, Madanes, Watzlawick and many others has been adequate to permit me to communicate about the kind of therapeutic relationship and approach to therapy that I think can make a difference in effecting therapeutic change. Although it is a relationship that is not necessary to every therapeutic situation, it is relevant to most with which I have been familiar. The peculiar form of this therapeutic relationship and the predictable sequences of communication which characterize it establishes an interpersonal context which comprises a fertile ground for change.

Yet, it is important to remember that the language used to describe the approach, such as "paradox" and other constructs specified here, is not essential to the approach. That is why diversity was important in the case examples used for illustration. The diversity consisted of problems of various kinds, various forms of therapy, and depictions which were both brief and detailed. With the succession of case illustrations, this diversity permitted the construction of a redundant and resonant convergence of ideas, consisting of a basic understanding about effecting therapeutic change, but an understanding that does not require adherence to, or reification of, any construct. I hope that it has been an explication which is clear and coherent enough to provide continuing guidance to myself and to any others who may find it of some use.

REFERENCES

Andreychuck, T., & Skriver, C. Hypnosis and biofeedback in the treatment of migraine headache. *International Journal of Clinical and Experimental Hypnosis*, 1975, *23*, 172-183.

Arnheim, R. *Visual thinking*. London: Faber and Faber Limited, 1969.

Atkinson, R.C., & Shiffrin, R.M. Human memory: a proposed system and its control process. In K. Spence and H. Spence (Eds.), *The psychology of learning and motivation in research and theory: Volume 2*. New York: Academic Press, 1968.

Bakan, P. Hypnotizability, laterality of eye movement and functional brain asymmetry. *Perceptual and Motor Skills*, 1969, *28*, 927-932.

Baker, E. L. The use of hypnotic dreaming in the treatment of the borderline patient: some thoughts on resistance and transitional phenomena. *The International Journal of Clinical Experimental Hypnosis*, 1983, *31*, 19-27.

Bandler, R., & Grinder, J. *Patterns of the hypnotic techniques of Milton H. Erickson, M.D.: Volume 1*. Cupertino, CA.: Meta Publications, 1975.

Barber, T. X., & Glass, L. B. Significant factors in hypnotic behavior. *Journal of Abnormal and Social Psychology*, 1962, *64*, 222-228.

Barber, T. X., & Calverley, D. S. An experimental study of "hypnotic" (auditory and visual) hallucinations. *Journal of Abnormal and Social Psychology*, 1964, *63*, 13-20.

Barber, T. X. *Hypnosis: a scientific approach*. New York: Van Nostrand Reinhold, 1969.

Barber, T. X., Spanos, N. P., & Chaves, J. F. *Hypnotism: imagination and human potentialities*. New York: Pergamon, 1974.

Bateson, G. *Steps to an ecology of mind*. San Francisco: Chandler, 1972.

Beck, A. T. *Depression: clinical, experimental and theoretical aspects*. New York: Harper and Row, 1967.

Binet, A., & Fere, C. *Animal magnetism*. New York: Appleton & Company, 1901.

Bopp, M. J., & Weeks, G. R. Dialectical metatheory in family therapy. *Family Process*, 1984, *23*, 49-62.

Bordin, E. S. The generalizability of the psychoanalytic concept of the working alliance. *Psychotherapy: Theory, research, and practice*, 1979, *16*, 252-260.

Boszormenyi-Nagy, I. A theory of relationships: Experience and transaction. In I. Boszormenyi-Nagy and J. Framo (Eds.), *Intensive family therapy: theoretical and practical aspects*. New York: Harper & Row, 1965.

Bowers, K. S. Hypnotic behavior: the differentiation of trance and demand characteristic variables. *Journal of Abnormal Psychology*, 1966, *71*, 42-51.

Bowers, K. S. *Hypnosis for the seriously curious*. Monterey, CA: Brooks/Cole, 1976.

Bowers, M., & Glasner, S. Autohypnotic aspects of the Jewish cabbalistic concept of kavana. *Journal of Clinical and Experimental Hypnosis*, 1958, *6*, 50.

Braid, J. *Neurypnology: or the rationale of nervous sleep*. 1843. Revised as *Braid on hypnotism*. New York: Julian Press, 1960.

Brooks, R. Creative characters: a technique in child therapy. *Psychotherapy: Theory, Research, & Practice*, 1981, *18*, 131-139.

Castaneda, C. *Journey to Ixtlan: The lessons of Don Juan*. New York: Simon & Schuster, 1972.

Craik, F. I., & Lockhart, R. S. Levels of processing: a framework for memory research. *Journal of Verbal Learning and Verbal Behavior*, 1972, *11*, 671-684.

Deikman, A. J. *The observing self*. Boston: Beacon Press, 1982.

Dell, P. Some irreverant thoughts on paradox. *Family Process*, 1981, *20*, 37-41.

Desoille, R. *The directed daydream*. New York: Psychosynthesis Research Foundation, 1966.

Didato, S. V. *Psychotechniques*. New York: Methuen, 1980.

Edmonston, W. E. Stimulus-response theory of hypnosis. In J. E. Gordon (Ed.), *Handbook of Clinical and Experimental Hypnosis*. New York: MacMillan Co., 1967.

Ellenberger, H. F. *The discovery of the unconscious: the history and evolution of dynamic psychiatry*. New York: Basic Books, 1970.

Ellis, A. *Reason and emotion in psychotherapy*. Secaucus, N. J.: The Citadel Press, 1977.

Elkaim, M. From general laws to singularities. *Family Process*, 1985, *24*, 151-164.

Elmore, A. M. A comparison of the psychophysiological and clinical response to biofeedback for temporal pulse amplitude reduction and biofeedback for increases in hand temperature in the treatment of migraine. Unpublished doctoral dissertation. State University of New York at Stoneybrook, 1979.

Erickson, M. H. *Healing in hypnosis: The seminars, workshops, and lectures of Milton H. Erickson - Volume 1*. New York: Irvington Publishers, 1983.

Erickson, M. H. *The collected papers of Milton H. Erikson on hypnosis: Volumes 1-4*. New York: Irvington Publishers, 1980.

Erickson, M. H., Rossi, E. L., & Rossi, S. I. *Hypnotic realities*. New York: Irvington, 1976.

Fahrion, S. L. Autogenic biofeedback treatment for migraine. *Mayo Clinic Procedures*, 1977, *52*, 776-784.

Ferenczi, S., & Rank. O. *The development of psychoanalysis*. New York: Dover, 1956.

Fisch, R., Weakland, J. H., & Segal, L. *The tactics of change: doing therapy briefly*. San Francisco: Jossey-Bass, 1982.

Fischer, C. Studies on the nature of suggestion. Part II: The transference meaning of giving suggestions. *Journal of the American Psychiatric Association,* 1953, *1,* 222-255.

Fogarty, T. Marital crisis. In P. J. Guerin (Ed.), *Family therapy: theory and practice.* New York: Gardner, 1976.

Freud, S. (1921), *Group psychology and the analysis of the ego.* London: Hogarth, 1955.

Freud, S. (1900), *Three essays on the theory of sexuality.* London: Hogarth, 1953.

Gardner, G. G., & Olness, K. *Hypnosis and hypnotherapy with children.* New York: Grune & Stratton, Inc., 1981.

Gardner, R. *Psychotherapeutic approaches to the resistant child.* New York: Aronson, 1975.

Gibson, H. B. *Hypnosis: its nature and therapeutic benefits.* London: Peter Owen, 1977.

Gibson, H. B. & Corcoran, M. E. Personality and differential susceptibility to hypnosis: further replication and sex differences. *British Journal of Psychology,* 1975, *66,* 513-520.

Gibson, H. B., & Curran, J. D. Hypnotic susceptibility and personality: a replication study. *British Journal of Psychology,* 1974, *65,* 283-291.

Gill, M. M., & Brenman, M. The metapsychology of regression and hypnosis. In J. E. Gordon (Ed.), *Handbook of Clinical and Experimental Hypnosis.* New York: MacMillan Co., 1967.

Gill, M. M., & Brenman, M. *Hypnosis and related states.* New York: International Universities Press, 1959.

Gilligan, S. G. Ericksonian approaches to clinical hypnosis. In J. K. Zeig (Ed.), *Ericksonian approaches to hypnosis and psychotherapy.* New York: Bruner/Mazel, 1982.

Ginott, H. G. *Between parent and child.* New York: Macmillan, 1965.

Glasner, S. A note on allusions to hypnosis in the Bible and Talmud. *Journal of Clinical and Experimental Hypnosis,* 1955, *3,* 34.

Gordon, T. *Parent effectiveness training in action.* New York: Wyden, 1976.

Gur, R. C., & Gur, R. E. Handedness, sex, and eyedness as moderating variables in the relation between hypnotic susceptibility and functional brain asymmetry. *Journal of Abnormal Psychology,* 1974, *83,* 635-643.

Haley, J. An interactional explanation of hypnosis. *The American Journal of Clinical Hypnosis,* 1958, *1,* 41-57.

Haley, J. *Strategies of psychotherapy.* New York: Grune & Stratton, 1963.

Haley, J. *Uncommon therapy.* New York: Balantine, 1974.

Haley, J. *Problem solving therapy: New strategies for effective family therapy.* San Francisco: Jossey-Bass, 1978.

Haley, J. *Ordeal therapy: Unusual ways to change behavior.* San Francisco: Jossey-Bass, 1984.

Hallaji, J. Hypnotherapeutic techniques in a Central Asian community, *The International Journal of Clinical and Experimental Hypnosis,* 1962, *10,* 271-274.

Haynes, J. M. *Divorce Mediation: A practical guide for therapists and counselors.* New York: Springer, 1981.

Hilgard, E. R. *Hypnotic susceptibility*. New York: Harcourt, Brace, and World, 1965.

Hilgard, E. R. A critique of Johnson, Maher, and Barber's 'Artifact in the essence of hypnosis': an evaluation of trance logic with a recomputation of their findings. *Journal of Abnormal Psychology*, 1972, *79*, 221-233.

Hilgard, E. R. A neodissociation interpretation of pain reduction in hypnosis. *Psychological Review*, 1973, *80*, 396-411. (a)

Hilgard, E. R. The domain of hypnosis, with some comments on alternative paradigms. *American Psychologist*, 1973, *28*, 972-982. (b)

Hilgard, E. R. Hypnosis. *Annual Review of Psychology*. 1975, *26*, 19-44.

Hilgard, J. R. Personality and hypnotizability: inferences from case studies. In E. R. Hilgard (Ed.), *Hypnotic susceptibility*. New York: Harcourt, Brace, & World, Inc.: 1965.

Hilgard, J. R. *Personality and hypnosis: A study of imaginative involvement.* Chicago: University of Chicago Press, 1970.

Hoffman, L. *Foundations of family therapy: A conceptual framework for systems change*. New York: Basic Books, 1981.

Hoorwitz, A. N. "Extraordinary circumstances" in custody contests between parent and non-parent. *Journal of Psychiatry and Law*, 1982, *10*, 351-361.

Hoorwitz, A. N. The visitation dilemma in court consultation. *Social Casework*, 1983, *64*, 231-237.

Hoorwitz, A. N. Establishing partial limits on children's behavior: Use of strategic, structural, and cognitive-behavioral approaches. *American Journal of Family Therapy*, 1985, *13*, 56-64.

Hoorwitz, A. N., & Burchardt, C. J. Procedures for court consultations on child custody issues. *Social Casework*, 1984, *65*, 259-266.

Hull, C. L. *Hypnosis and suggestibility: an experimental approach*. New York: Appleton-Century-Crofts, 1933.

Hunt, S. M. Hypnosis as obedience behavior. *British Journal of Social and Clinical Psychology*, 1979, *18*, 21-27.

Hutt, L. Interpretation and hope. *Psychotherapy: Theory, research, and practice*, 1976, *13*, 259-262.

Hynan, M. T. On the advantages of assuming that the techniques of psychotherapy are ineffective. *Psychotherapy: Theory, research, and practice*, 1981, *18*, 11-13.

Johnson, R. F., Maher, B. A., & Barber, T. X. Artifact in the 'essence of hypnosis': an evaluation of trance logic. *Journal of Abnormal Psychology*, 1972, *79*, 212-220.

Kaplan, H. S. *The new sex therapy*. New York: Bruner/Mazel, 1974.

Kroger, W. S. *Clinical and experimental hypnosis in medicine, dentistry, and psychology (2nd edition)*. Philadelphia: J. B. Lippincott Company, 1977.

Kubie, L. S., & Margolin, S. The process of hypnotism and the nature of the hypnotic state. *The American Journal of Psychiatry*, 1944, *100*, 611-622.

Lang, P. J., & Lazowik, A. D. Personality and hypnotic susceptibility. *Journal of Consulting Psychology*, 1962, *26*, 317-333.

Lankton, S. R., & Lankton, C. H. *The answer within: a clinical framework of Ericksonian hypnotherapy*. New York: Bruner/Mazel, 1983.

Lazarus, A. *In the mind's eye: the power of imagery for personal enrichment.* New York: Rawson Associates Publishers, Inc., 1977.

Levitt, E. E., & Baker, E. L. The hypnotic relationship - another look at coercion, compliance and resistance: a brief communication. *The International Journal of Clinical and Experimental Hypnosis,* 1983, *31,* 125-131.

Lindner, H. The shared neurosis: hypnotist and subject. *International Journal of Clinical Hypnosis,* 1960, *8,* 61-70.

London, P. Ethics in hypnosis. In J. E. Gordon (Ed.), *Handbook of Clinical and Experimental Hypnosis.* New York: Macmillan Co., 1967.

Madanes, C. *Strategic Family Therapy.* San Francisco: Jossey-Bass, 1981.

Masters, W. H., & Johnson, V. E. *Human sexual response.* Boston: Little, Brown, 1966.

Masters, W. H., & Johnson, V. E. *Human sexual inadequacy.* Boston: Little, Brown, 1970.

Minuchin, S. *Families and family therapy.* Cambridge, MA: Harvard University Press, 1974.

Mullinex, J. M., Norton, B. J., Hack, S., & Fishman, M. A. Skin temperature, biofeedback and migraine. *Headache,* 1978, *17,* 242-244.

O'Connor, J. The resurrection of a magical reality: treatment of functional migraine in a child. *Family Process,* 1984, *23,* 501-509.

O'Connor, J. J. Strategic psychotherapy. In I. Kutash and A. Wolf (Eds.), *Psychotherapist's casebook: theory and technique in practice.* San Francisco: Jossey-Bass, 1985.

O'Connor, J., & Hoorwitz, A. N. The bogeyman cometh: a strategic approach for difficult adolescents. *Family Process,* 1984, *23,* 237-249.

Orne, M. T. The nature of hypnosis: artifact and essence. *The Journal of Abnormal and Social Psychology,* 1966, *58,* 277-299.

Orne, M. T. Hypnosis, motivation, and compliance. *American Journal of Psychiatry,* 1966, *122,* 721-726.

Orne, M. T. Can a hypnotized subject be compelled to carry out otherwise unacceptable behavior? *International Journal of Clinical and Experimental Hypnosis,* 1972, *20,* 107.

Palazzoli, M. S., Boscolo, L., Cecchin, G., & Prata, G. *Paradox and counterparadox.* New York: Jason Aronson, 1978.

Papp, P. The Greek chorus and other techniques of family therapy. *Family Process,* 1980, *19,* 45-57.

Pardell, S. S. Psychology of the hypnotist. *Psychiatric Quarterly,* 1950, *24,* 483-491.

Phillips, D., & Judd, R. *How to fall out of love.* Boston: Houghton Mifflin, 1978.

Ritterman, M. K. Hemophilia in context: adjunctive hypnosis for families with a hemophiliac member. *Family Process,* 1982, *21,* 469-476.

Rosen, S. *My voice will go with you: the teaching tales of Milton H. Erickson.* New York: Norton, 1982.

Sarbin, T. R. Contributions to role-taking theory: Hypnotic behavior. *Psychological Review,* 1950, *57,* 255-270.

Sarbin, T. R., & Anderson, M. L. Role-theoretical analysis of hypnotic behavior.

In J. E. Gordon (Ed.), *Handbook of clinical and experimental hypnosis*. New York: Macmillan Company, 1967.

Sarbin, T. R., & Coe, W. C. *Hypnosis: a social psychological analysis of influence communication*. New York: Holt, Rinehart, & Winston, 1972.

Sarbin, R. T., & Lim, D. T. Some evidence in support of the role-taking hypothesis in hypnosis. *International Journal of Clinical and Experimental Hypnosis*, 1963, *11*, 98-103.

Sargent, J. D., Green, E. E., & Walters, E. D. Preliminary report on the use of autogenic feedback training in the treatment of migraine and tension headaches. *Psychosomatic Medicine*, 1973, *35*, 129-235.

Schilder, P., & Kauders, O. A textbook of hypnosis. In P. Schilder (Ed.), *The nature of hypnosis*. New York: International Universities Press, 1956.

Sheehan, P. W., & Perry, C. W. *Methodologies of hypnosis: a critical appraisal of contemporary paradigms of hypnosis*. Hillsdale, N.J.: Laurence Erlbaum, 1976.

Shor, R. E. Hypnosis and the concept of the generalized reality-orientation. *American Journal of Psychotherapy*, 1959, *13*, 582-602.

Shor, R. E., & Orne, M. T. (Eds.), *The nature of hypnosis: selected basic readings*. New York: Holt, Rinehart, & Winston, Inc., 1965.

Spanos,N. P., & Barber, T. X. Toward a convergence in hypnosis research. *American Psychologist*, 1974, *29*, 500-511.

Spiegel, H. A single treatment method to stop smoking using ancillary self hypnosis. *International Journal of Clinical and Experimental Hypnosis*, 1970, *18*, 235-250.

Stanton, M. D. Fusion, compression, diversion, and the working of paradox: a theory of therapeutic/systemic change. *Family Process*, 1984, *23*, 135-167.

Starker, S. Effects of hypnotic induction upon visual imagery. *Journal of Nervous and Mental Disease*, 1974, *159*, 433-437.

Sutcliffe, J. P. "Credulous" and "skeptical" views of hypnotic phenomena: a review of certain evidence and methodology. *International Journal of Clinical and Experimental Hypnosis*, 1960, *8*, 73-101.

Sutcliffe, J. P. "Credulous" and "skeptical" views of hypnotic phenomena: experiments on esthesia, hallucination, and delusion. *Journal of Abnormal and Social Psychology*, 1961, *62*, 189-200.

Thornton, E. M. *Hypnotism, hysteria, and epilepsy: an historical synthesis*. London: Heinemann, 1976.

Tinterow, M. M. *Foundations of hypnosis: from Mesmer to Freud*. Springfield, Ill.: Charles C. Thomas, 1970.

Torrey, E. F. What Western psychotherapists can learn from witchdoctors. *American Journal of Orthopsychiatry*, 1972, *42*, 67-76.

Wagstaff, G. F. *Hypnosis, compliance, and belief*, New York: St. Martin's Press, 1981.

Watkins, M. Concept and measurement of primary memory. *Psychological Bulletin*, 1974, *81*, 695-711.

Weeks, G. R., & L'Abate, L. *Paradoxical psychotherapy: Theory and practice with individuals, couples, and families*. New York: Bruner/Mazel, 1982.

Weitzenhoffer, A. M., & Hilgard, E. R. *Stanford hypnotic susceptibility scale, forms A and B*. Palo Alto, CA: Consulting Psychologists Press, 1959.

White, R. W. Two types of hypnotic trance and their personality correlates. *The Journal of Psychology*, 1937, *3*, 279-289.

White, R. W. A preface to the theory of hypnotism. *Journal of Abnormal and Social Psychology*, 1941, *36*, 477-505.

Witmer, L. The use of hypnotism in education. *Pediatrics*, 1897, *3*, 23-27.

Zeig, J. K. *Teaching Seminar with Milton H. Erickson, M.D.* New York: Bruner/Mazel, 1980.

Zeig, J. K. *Ericksonian approaches to hypnosis and psychotherapy*. New York: Bruner/Mazel, 1982.

INDEX